Contents

KU-647-677

0121613

Issues in
GENERAL ED

Educating for Health

JKT HH
(1ku)

0304328022

Other books in this series

Michael Barber: Education and the Teacher Unions

Gordon Batho: Political Issues in Education

David Bosworth: Open Learning

Paul Fisher: Education 2000

Eric Hoyle and Peter D. John: Professional Knowledge and
Professional Practice

Roy Todd: Education in a Multicultural Society

Geoffrey Walford: Choice and Equity in Education

Michael Williams: In-Service Education and Training

Leo B. Hendry, Janet Shucksmith and
Kate Philip

Educating for Health

School and Community Approaches with Adolescents

CASSELL

Cassell
Wellington House
125 Strand
London WC2R 0BB

215 Park Avenue South
New York
NY 10003

British Library Cataloguing in Publication Data
A catalogue record for this book is available from the British Library

ISBN 0–304–32804–9 (hardback)
     0–304–32802–2 (paperback)

Typeset by Action Typesetting Limited, Gloucester
Printed and bound in Great Britain by Biddles Ltd, Guildford, Surrey

Foreword: the purpose of this series

The educational scene is changing rapidly. This change is being caused by a complexity of factors which includes a re-examination of present educational provision against a background of changing social and economic policies, new forms of testing and assessment, a National Curriculum, and local management of schools with more participation by parents.

As the educational process is concerned with every aspect of our lives and our society both now and for the future, it is of vital importance that all teachers, teachers in training, administrators and educational policy-makers should be aware and informed on current issues in education.

This series of books is thus designed to inform on current issues, to look at emerging ones, and to give an authoritative overview which will be of immense help to all those involved in the education process.

Philip Hills
Cambridge

Preface

In researching many aspects of young people's lifestyles and health dilemmas in the last fifteen years we have often felt inclined to paraphrase the saying that 'youth is wasted on the young' to say instead that 'health is wasted on the young'.

Characteristically, we value least what we have the most of. The young seem to have health and vigour in abundance. But many of them appear to do their best to squander it or jeopardize it by adopting health-threatening behaviours such as smoking or drug misuse.

Part of their nonchalance in the face of the frustration of their elders is, perhaps, due to their inability to visualize life for themselves twenty or thirty years down the road. Elkind's (1985) characterization of the 'personal fable' (used to explain risk-taking behaviour) serves as well to describe activities like poor dietary habits, for example, which, while not outrageously risky in the short-term, clearly have long-term consequences for young people's health.

Are young people, though, really any more irrational than the older members of society? Every day even the oldest and wisest of us ignore good advice, though well aware of the likely consequences of our actions. We must beware of caricaturing youth as unremittingly feckless. The first section of this book addresses itself to the question of whether adolescence as a stage of life really does have distinctive characteristics, and then goes on to examine whether these are associated with a particular range of health issues or problems.

Are there issues relating to the way young people consider their health that have an impact on the way education programmes are offered? A strong theme of the book is that consideration needs to be given to the belief and value systems of young people in the context of the sub-cultures in which they live. This raises the important question of how to take account of the young person's perspective within the health domain. We believe strongly that a 'collaborative' approach to health education is vital in order to enhance adolescents' transition to adulthood, and we explore this statement and its implications for both school and community settings.

If this approach seems somewhat challenging we would point both to high levels of dissatisfaction with the effectiveness of much past and recent health education work with young people and also to a groundswell of change in the way in which young people are viewed and treated, amounting almost to a paradigm shift. The Children Act (HMSO, 1989), for instance, has set in motion a range of recommendations giving young people greater rights within society – in the family, at school, in the wider community, and in relation to their health care. The call for 'rights of citizenship' for youth has also resounded in a number of recent academic texts (Coleman and Warren-Adamson, 1992; Jones and Wallace, 1992). Thus what we are exploring here offers a contribution to a new paradigm for both theoretical and policy debates about young people's health. Unlike other health models, our framework takes account of the idea of adolescents' self-agency within the socialization process (Lerner, 1985; Coleman and Hendry, 1990) and extends this through into the field of health. Thus we provide a different way of approaching adolescent health concerns, health education and health promotion.

In Chapters 3 to 6 then, this book sets out to explore issues in health education and health promotion in the context of both schools and the wider community. The book does not pretend to be a comprehensive survey of health education approaches, nor does it provide an outline curriculum in health education. It is not intended to be a 'recipe book' of health and health education for teachers and other professionals. Rather,

within the text we raise a number of key issues in health education by taking a variety of theoretical models, research
findings, examples and case studies in order to illuminate
aspects of young people's health needs, their learning capacity
and ways of acquiring knowledge and behaviours in the health
domain. A consideration of what adult society provides
through its education institutions is also undertaken and we
examine a number of pertinent professional concerns in school
and community settings. The overarching question addressed
in the book is how different perspectives can be 'married'
together in order to develop health education meaningfully in
school and community in a manner that enables young people's
concerns to be addressed and in turn empowers them to make a
successful transition towards adulthood, powerfully aided and
abetted by the professional workers, and other adults, who
have a commitment to young people's health. Thus the book
attempts to look at issues around the theme of linking adult
concerns about young people's health with the adolescents'
own perspective.

Importantly, we reflect on the issues of health concerns,
'interventions' and research – most of which emanates from an
adultist perspective – by trying to 'redress the balance' and
thereby including ideas and findings which offer young
people's views on health and health education.

Our own research into youth health issues in the past ten
years or so has included a seven-year longitudinal project –
part survey, part illuminative – of 10,000 young people's
developing lifestyles; an ethnographic interview study of
adolescents in relation to HIV/AIDS, drugs and sexual relationships; an examination and review of information and
drop-in centres for young people using case study methods; an
action research project exploring young people's ability to
become peer educators within their own communities; and a
development project working with teachers and community
educators on health topics. We have thus gleaned the views
and perspectives of young people and the professionals and
other adults who work with them on health issues through a

variety of different methods.

The settings for these studies have been urban and rural communities throughout Scotland. However, while our own empirical focus has largely been Scottish, this book incorporates research findings from all parts of the United Kingdom, and from further afield, and the interpretations, theoretical frameworks and general principles which emerge from our writings are applicable from Land's End to John O'Groats for those who work with young people, or are studying for health care or social service professions, or are simply interested in young people's development.

In the first chapter of this book, we explore aspects of the adolescent transition together with some of the attendant health issues and concerns. The second chapter considers research findings about young people's health within a British context and discusses issues in both questionnaire survey and illuminative case study approaches.

Chapters 3 and 4 consider health education in schools and how school health education curricula have developed in response to prevailing paradigms incorporating views about learning and rationality. Chapter 3 discusses whether schools provide appropriate settings for eliciting young people's needs and beliefs. The implication of more collaborative modes of working brings us to a discussion of empowerment and to the debate about whether a health education curriculum developed along these lines would be highly dissonant with the prevailing ethos of the modern school. Chapter 4 explores some of the professional dilemmas facing teachers on the ground with respect to the demands made upon them to develop innovative and radical health education agendas. Development work from our own study of teachers exploring issues around the development of a syllabus to educate about sexual behaviour is used as a case study to illustrate some of the unsolved problems now facing schools as they get caught 'between the devil and the deep blue sea', trying to respond to young people's needs and trying to keep the other participants in the educational enterprise happy too.

Chapters 5 and 6 consider adolescent health in a community context and look at a variety of theoretical models and professional approaches which go some way to addressing the heterogeneity of youth. Chapter 6 in particular looks at specific examples of youth work interventions, such as peer tutoring and outreach work, and discusses how far these radical methods can help community workers address health issues with young people.

The final chapter of the book attempts to draw together the themes and issues presented throughout the text and re-examines the intriguing question of young people's rights and our responsibilities as parents and educators. Pressure mounts on the countries of the developed world to implement the United Nations Charter on the Rights of the Child. How has this issue been addressed to date, and what are the implications in terms of health education of adapting an approach which puts the child at the centre rather than at the periphery of the decision-making process?

1   Being young, growing up

Introduction

Young people are never far from the headlines in today's press, but the ambivalence with which we view them is well summed up in a small selection of recent banners. Are they, for instance, the source of trouble, ('Children's lazy life puts nation's health at risk', *Sunday Times*, 16 January 1994), or merely the innocent victims of others' neglect at a personal or structural level ('The family at war', *Sunday Times*, 7 March 1993; 'Parents blamed for stressed out teens', *Sunday Times*, 12 July 1994)?

Do such headlines reflect the issues facing adolescents growing up today and accurately highlight society's concerns for their general well-being? Or are they themes which have re-emerged at regular intervals throughout history? Davis (1990) has shown, by tracing historically the general public 'images' of adolescents in society, that themes of rebellion, moodiness and 'angst', deliquency, 'sinfulness', energy, excitement and idealistic views of future society have been retained in adults' consciousness, and reinforced by the mass media, thus creating stereotypic pictures of youth in Britain today. Davis has traced the history of notions like 'youth as national (economic) asset', 'youth as minority stereotype' (positive as well as negative) and 'youth as a litmus test' (of the good and ills of the society). He demonstrates how these, though waxing and waning, have all (sometimes simultaneously) been key themes in the history of the concept of youth. He also documents how, alongside all this, and especially from the

1

1960s onwards, a 'youth culturalisation' of mainstream adult life has taken place. What makes this even more paradoxical is Davis's central theme: 'youth as continuity'. For he, like many others before him, provides ample evidence that, far from being revolutionary or even passively subversive, young people have, over many generations, been deeply committed to the basic values and institutions of their society. The problem (especially for them) has been that adult power-holders have needed to construct images and to accumulate 'data' which 'prove' the opposite in order to justify their requirement for controlling and for offering highly oppressive responses to youth. Such controls may operate differently for young men and young women. Young women, for instance, may face contradictory sets of expectations in school (Stanworth, 1983) and in wider society (McRobbie, 1991) and be 'offered' particular role models by the media (Scraton, 1986).

What is adolescence? While this is an important question to ask, the answer is not a simple one. In the first place no one is entirely sure when this transitional stage from childhood to adulthood begins. For some it may be at 13 years, the first 'teen' year, while for others it may be at the start of secondary school. For those who prefer a physical marker the commencement of puberty is the obvious moment, yet puberty itself is a very complex phenomenon, with different elements – the growth spurt, menarche, and so on – occurring at different times. The picture is further confused by the fact that, during the twentieth century in western industrialized countries, menarche has occurred approximately one month earlier every decade of the century (Coleman and Hendry, 1990). Today a proportion of girls in the top class of any primary school will have started puberty – are these 10- or 11-year-olds adolescent? The situation is even more confused at the upper end of the age range. If legal definitions are to be relied upon one is adult in some respects at 16, in other respects at 17, and yet others at 18 years. Continued education and training after 16 years of age for many in our society lead to prolonged dependence on the family. Adulthood is postponed, and more and more young people remain at home until their early twenties. A startling statistic is that in Britain the average age for leaving home in 1979 was 19. In 1990 it was 23! (Griffin, 1992). These social shifts have been a result of radical changes in social policy and practice towards young people (and their families) which have moved some of the financial onus for support from the state to individuals and families (Coleman and Warren-Adamson, 1992).

Adolescent development emerges from an interaction among the socialization processes of childhood, physical maturation, the socio-cultural pressures associated with adolescence itself and the active self-agency of the individual. New social situations and the demands they present are likely to encourage the development of additional personal resources and skills. Nevertheless on certain occasions particular patterns of social response may be called for and the skills necessary may not have yet developed in the young (Furnham, 1986; Rutter, 1989). The nature and type of these responses may have important consequences for future patterns of behaviour and for the adolescent's self-perceptions and feelings of self-efficacy (Bandura, 1981). This means that the pathway which an individual adolescent takes towards adulthood may be quite different from the pathways followed by his or her peers (Roberts and Parsell, 1989; Rutter, 1989; Wallace, 1989). We must also remember that the various transitions of adolescence occur when many parents are approaching their own mid-life concerns, crises and changes in their life course (Sheehy, 1976). These parental effects can 'interact' with the adolescent's own efforts to develop self-esteem and self-efficacy in ways that are less than optimal for development and psycho-social growth.

One certainty is that in youthful populations good health is apparently the norm. However, while adolescence is in general a healthy stage of the lifespan, it may be the genesis of behaviour patterns which are carried into adulthood with possible health risks. There seems little doubt that some of the most important events to which young people have to adjust are the multitude of physiological and bodily changes which occur during early adolescence and which are associated with what is generally known as puberty. Sexual maturation is closely linked to those physical changes, and the sequence of events is approximately 18 to 24 months later for boys than it is for girls. Such changes inevitably exercise a profound effect upon the individual. The body alters radically in size and shape, and it is not surprising that many adolescents experience a period of clumsiness as they attempt to adapt to these changes. The body also alters in function, and new and sometimes worrying physical experiences such as the girl's first period, or the boy's nocturnal emissions, have to be understood. Perhaps most important of all, however, is the effect that such physical changes have upon identity. As many writers have pointed out, the development of the individual's identity requires not only the notion of being separate and different from others, but also a sense of self-consistence, and a firm knowledge of how one appears to the rest of the world. Needless to say dramatic bodily changes seriously affect these aspects of identity, and also represent a considerable challenge in adaptation for even the most well-adjusted young person, especially since such changes may cause others to have altered expectations for the adolescent.

In this chapter we examine briefly whether adolescence is a very different experience for today's young people. What features of the social and cultural context might make the adolescent transition more difficult to manoeuvre?

We move on from here to examine in some depth the features of change which research has traditionally explored in adolescence. Physical changes as young people approach puberty and pass through it are the most visible signs of change, but other critical areas are those of the developing self-identity of the young person and also the development of social and relational understanding.

These physical, psychological and social changes are described in order to paint a backdrop about adolescence in which we hope to contextualize our discussion about health education.

We conclude this chapter by looking at how all of these three levels of change are implicated in the putative association between young people and risk-taking. We ask whether young people really are particularly prone to taking risks, explore whether there is a positive as well as a negative side to their risk-taking behaviour and then examine how risk-taking is associated with a variety of health issues.

Changing times for adolescents?

One of the most striking findings from recent research is the essentially conventional nature of the majority of young people (Davis, 1990; Hendry *et al.*, 1993b). Most recent findings have also noted the increasingly fragmentary nature of youth groups breaking down the notion of some unifying youth culture (Brake, 1980). Hendry *et al.* have demonstrated the variety of pathways which occur within and across social class boundaries as young people's lifestyles develop within the adolescent years. However, the way young people view themselves and their attitudes needs to be seen against a wider picture of essentially material and consumer-led aspirations (Gardner and Sheppard, 1989). Currently there are about four million 15- to 19-year olds and about four and a half million 20- to 24-year-olds in the United Kingdom. Together they comprise almost 15 per cent of the population. Given the increasingly consumer-oriented nature of the society we inhabit, commercial influences on young people's lives have grown and these have had, and are having, a profound impact on adolescence and young people. It is clear, for instance, that young people are becoming active in adult commercial markets at even younger ages. A survey by the British Market Research Bureau (1990) asked young people how they would spend a hypothetical £50. Teenagers within this group were most interested in spending on clothes, records, tapes and cosmetics, while those in their early twenties were more likely to spend their money on entertainments or to save up for specific consumer items. There also appears to be a close correlation between the way young people spend their leisure time and their expenditure priorities. A major factor that has important implications for leisure time use is mobility. Here it is significant to note that one third of those in their early twenties drives a car or van on a regular basis (Stewart, 1992).

Many would claim that despite growing affluence in the industrialized nations (or perhaps because of it) the social expectations for youth are even more problematic than in previous eras. As society has become more diverse and complex the number of social roles and choices facing teenagers has altered dramatically. The ways in which young people select among these roles and lifestyles is harder to predict because political and moral values have become more diverse as we have moved to a pluralistic post-modern society. There is an element of freedom in this variety, but 'freedom' for adolescents carries with it risks and one can enumerate the costs of making errors in judgement: 'dropping out' of school, being out of work, teenage pregnancy, sexually transmitted diseases, being homeless, drug addiction and suicide are powerful examples of the price that some young people pay for making inappropriate choices. The impact of making 'wrong' choices on individuals, families and wider society underscores the need for a better understanding of adolescent development and the transition to adulthood.

Government legislation and policy concerning education, occupational training, social benefits and other aspects of youth's transition to adulthood create a longer period of dependency on the family – or state – for material support and marginalize young people from society because they are expected to be adults but are not given commensurate responsibility (Jones and Wallace, 1992), nor included as genuine partners with adults in collaborative ventures in work or at lesiure (Love and Hendry, 1994).

Young people enter adolesence having been shaped by their biological and psychological characteristics and their earlier social experiences. Taken together, the experience of the younger child and of the adolescent are the mould from which the adult emerges. Social shifts have created new constraints, experiences and opportunities for adolescents, in a context where even well-established social institutions can be subject to change. The nuclear family is now juxtaposed with 'reconstituted' families, shared child-custody arrangements and single-parent homes. Additionally changes in social attitudes towards, and expectations for, adolescents have occurred in many spheres of life. To cite two examples: access to illicit drugs is now a common feature of growing up for many young people; and the transition from school to full-time employment is highly problematic at the present time. The erosion of the traditional roles of the family, the church and the school – institutions originally associated with socialization of the young – has resulted in the fragmentation of the adolescent transition since various social environments function as independent, sometimes isolated, and at times competitive or even contradictory settings for teenagers. It is this confusion of purpose at the community level and the disaffections which young people may develop towards it rather than any nationwide rebelliousness towards adult society which creates the possible conflicts of the adolescent identity crisis so frequently cited in the media. If the values expressed by different institutions are at odds, if their directions are unclear or inconsistent, the young person will be left with an uncertain set of guiding principles. Teenagers need to learn and express societal standards and expectations, not simply as sanctioned rules but as a loose collection of shared understandings which operate to limit the variability of acceptable behaviour.

Paradoxically, adolescents are too often described as passive recipients of circumstances and resources that other people make available to them. In reality, however, young people play an active role in choosing and shaping the context in which they operate and develop friendships, activities and lifestyles. The desires of parents and society at large to provide environments that promote 'acceptable' development might be simplified if we could gain a clearer understanding of why and how teenagers either resist or co-operate with such efforts

7

from adult society. For example, why do some adolescents function successfully as adults despite having grown up in adverse circumstances and contexts which are associated with generally negative outcomes? Conversely, why do others struggle to achieve adjustment despite coming from settings that seem to offer every advantage?

Recent debates concerning the dominant values operating in society; consumerism; the state of the family and schooling; the training and employment landscape facing adolescents; rising homelessness; teenage pregnancies; drugs; the threat of AIDS; crime and lawlessness bring into focus reflections of the adult world that young people face in the transition across adolescence.

In present-day society a number of adolescents and adults are more or less permanently excluded from full participation in the labour market in all industrialized societies. Furthermore, the probability of a given individual entering this section of the population underclass depends very much on his or her early labour market experiences. This is because much of what happens here has a self-reinforcing character. For example, the longer a spell of unemployment lasts, the lower the probability of the unemployed person finding a job. Or, to give another example, a 'poor' labour market record affords access to, at best, only unstable employment, attached to which is a high risk of unemployment and a further worsening of the individual's labour market position. We can, therefore, conceive of young people following particular labour market trajectories or being placed on particular 'paths', some of which lead to near permanent exclusion from the labour market.

Coffield *et al.* (1986) have drawn attention to the social circumstances of the individual young person, for these will obviously contribute in a substantial way to each adolescent's psychological adjustment. Gaining independence from parents has sociological and financial implications – as in unemployment – as well as being a psychological issue. There can be little doubt that in situations of economic hardship it will be more difficult to manage the adolescent transitions in a satisfactory manner:

> When a boy or girl personally accepts the label unemployed, the subjective environment changes. It becomes a state of inactivity and lassitude where personal powers cannot adequately be used or expressed. (Kitwood, 1980, pp.238–39)

It is certainly true that variations in the 'education-training-work-unemployment' patterns have become clearly embedded in the social landscape of the late 1980s and early 1990s. Thus youth unemployment has become an accepted – if not an acceptable – part of the transition to adulthood. Hendry (1983) mapped out a theoretical model of young people's leisure which envisaged a gradual transition across the teenage years from involvement in organized structured activities (in uniform groups and youth clubs) at age 11 to 13 through a period of mid-adolescence where casual activities with groups of peers were most valued (hanging about in the street, skateboarding at drop-in centres) at age 14 to 16 to a period in late adolescence when the peer group gives way to the courting dyad and when commercial leisure provision (pubs, clubs, discos) becomes available and irresistible. These leisure transitions coincide with Coleman's (1979) relational concerns. Recent empirical evidence (Hendry *et al.*, 1993a) confirms these theories. Thus, like Coleman's (1979) theory of adolescent focal issues, the reality of the process of unemployment can be viewed as a series of different psychological and social issues hitting the individual sequentially. Problems occur when several issues overlap. These factors in combination produce the elements around which coping strategies develop or a growing state of distress and poor mental health status emerges in the face of unemployment (Hendry and Raymond, 1986). The passage to adulthood for young unemployed without the resources to buy into a 'leisure package' in which many of the rituals of transition are enacted is a difficult one. Government attitudes to youth seem set to disadvantage adolescents even further. Attempts to turn round the welfare

9

philosophy that dominated post-war thinking will have an impact on young people at all levels of society. The withdrawal of benefits and grants ensures that parents remain responsible and young people remain dependent over a longer period of adolescence. Youth policy in the UK seems to have been constructed more to meet the needs of adult society than of young people (Coleman and Warren-Adamson, 1992).

Physical maturation

Much of the earlier work on physical maturation was concerned with mapping the timing of the different physical changes associated with puberty (Tanner, 1962) and with examining the psychological effects of early or late pubertal change (Davies, 1977). More recent work has tended to focus on the relationship between the biological changes of adolescence and other areas of development such as self-perception, social relations and social behaviour. Stattin and Magnusson (1990) have commented on the effects of maturational timing on young girls. Early maturers reported weight problems and expressed dissatisfaction with their temperament. Early developers also reported more problems in relationships with their parents, especially with mothers and with adult authority figures such as teachers. Such problems tended to be initiated by the young women rather than by the adults involved. Expectations held about early maturers as being 'more mature' may be interpreted with some confusion by such young people. In addition, they may quickly outgrow their peers socially. Timing of maturation was also noted in these studies to be related to patterns of social relationships. Early developers, for instance, preferred to associate with other early developers and late with late. Early maturers associated with older boys, were exposed to sexual experience at a younger age than other girls and were more likely to have had an abortion during the teenage years. Like Stattin and Magnusson, Silbereisen and Noack (1990) have examined the relationship between maturational timing and the varied aspects of psychological development with young men as well as young women. This study extended the earlier work by going beyond an analysis of the consequences of maturational timing for self-perception and for social relationships with parents and with other adolescents to look also at the links between maturational timing and involvement in problem behaviours such as smoking or under-age drinking. Their results suggested that early maturation has different effects on young men than on young women. With young men the effect is more likely to be positive, but for adolescent young women the opposite is true. Early maturing adolescent young women are more likely to associate with older males, to be unpopular with female age mates and to use cigarettes and alcohol to excess. Similarly late maturers, both young men and young women, were likely to be at a disadvantage in comparison with on time adolescents in a wide range of areas of development.

Rodriguez-Tomé and Bariaud (1990) have focused on three main areas of psychological development in relation to biological development during early adolescence, namely: cognitive processes, self-concept and socio-emotional reactions. Preliminary analyses have indicated that as maturation progresses young women evaluate their physical attractiveness but not their physical condition more negatively than young men. Young men's evaluation of their relationships with young women improves with physical maturation whereas girls' evaluation of relationships with young men remains more or less constant throughout the maturational period.

Experimental evidence has clearly shown that the average adolescent is not only sensitive to, but often critical of, his or her changing self (Clausen, 1975; Davies and Furnham, 1986). Perhaps as a result of media images and societal role models, teenagers tend to have idealized norms for physical attractiveness, and to feel inadequate if they do not match these unrealistic criteria. Lerner and Karabenick (1974) showed that adolescents who perceived themselves as deviating physically from cultural stereotypes were likely to have impaired self-concepts, and many other studies have pointed out the

11

important role that physical characteristics play in determining self-esteem, especially in the younger adolescent. Thus, for example, Rosen and Ross (1968), Simmons and Rosenberg (1975) and Hendry *et al.* (1993b) have reported studies in which adolescents were asked what they did and did not like about themselves. Results showed that those in early adolescence used primarily physical characteristics to describe themselves, and it was these characteristics which were most often disliked. It was not until later adolescence that intellectual or social aspects of personality were widely used in self-description, but these characteristics were much more frequently liked than disliked. It is just at the time of most rapid physical change that appearance is of critical importance for the individual, both for his or her self-esteem as well as for popularity with peers.

Self-identity and socialization

Beyond physical development and the accompanying growth and change of physical self-image, general self-concept and identity are important aspects of adolescence. Work aimed at defining the identity status of the individual stems from studies by Erikson (1968) who theorized that adolescence is characterized by an identity crisis (for an account of identity crises see Kroger, 1989). Within this field of study Marcia (1980) has set out to define identity formation behaviourally in terms of the achievement of commitments in late adolescence and the amount of exploration involved in this process. Bosma (1992) has extended the scope of Marcia's work to take more account of developmental change and of additional areas of commitment and exploration. Using a sample of young people aged 12 to 18 years Streitmatter (1985) examined differences in identity perceptions across age groups. The results of her study revealed indirect support for Erikson's speculations about the importance of this as an issue. The pattern found by Streitmatter indicated that male and female gender identification prior to adolescence was fairly distinct. Entry into adolescence seemed to cloud the issue. The pattern indicated decreasing differentiation from 12 and 13 to 14 years and from 14 to 15 years. However, 15– to 16–year-old comparisons reflected increasing differentiation. Apparently gender identifications which are adopted in childhood are reconsidered and reformulated during adolescence. Gilligan (1990) contended that as girls enter adolescence they seriously confront the disadvantages of their gender and suffer from an initial lack of confidence and a confused sense of identity. A second watershed appears to be the transition from school to work if, and when, girls discover how limited their occupational prospects are in contrast to boys – despite perhaps having achieved better grades at school – and they begin to have to make hard choices about career and personal life.

Using the social cognitive approaches Oosterwegel and Oppenheimer (1990) have distinguished between different features of self-concept such as actual self and ideal self and explored how these develop through childhood and adolescence, while Rodriguez-Tomé and Bariaud (1984) have shown that self-conceptions comprise more and more psychological and social interactional characteristics with increasing age. Other work has concentrated on the stability rather than the content of self-concepts. The results indicate that both self-concept and self-esteem remain fairly stable during adolescence and provide little evidence that adolescence is experienced as a stressful period (Fend, 1990; Coleman and Hendry, 1990). Social identity theory (Tajfel, 1982) emphasizes the link between the social and the personal aspects of identity. Clearly entry into a new phase in the life course challenges self-identity and particularly individual self-evaluations as young people attempt new tasks in which they can succeed or fail, as they alter their values and the areas which are important for overall self-esteem and as they confront new significant others against whom they rate themselves and about whose judgements they care. Rosenberg (1979) has emphasized the importance of the reflected self and of social comparison in determining self-esteem as well as the importance of doing

13

well in the areas one values (his principle of psychological centrality).

During adolescence clear changes take place in relationship patterns. Greater significance is given to peers as companions, as providers of advice, support and feedback, as models for behaviour and as sources of comparative information concerning personal qualities and skills. Relationships with parents alter in the direction of greater equality and reciprocity (Coleman and Hendry, 1990; Hendry *et al.*, 1993b) and parental authority comes to be seen as an area which is itself open to discussion and negotiation (Youniss and Smollar, 1990) and within which discriminations can be made (Coleman and Coleman, 1984). Fend (1990) investigated the relationship between ego strength development and social relationships, and showed that a decline in ego strength over time is related to a growing social gap between parents and peers. He also showed that the parent/adolescent relationship is more important than peer relationships for ego strength development. However, both types of relationship are of importance for coping successfully with the developmental tasks of adolescents in that both contribute to a positive self-concept. The significance of both types of relationships is supported by research carried out by Palmonari *et al.* (1989). Part of this work involved examining how Italian adolescents use different relationships in order to deal with various types of problems they encounter. A traditional (storm and stress) model would predict a straightforward change from 'reference to parents' to 'reference to peers' as adolescence progresses. In fact, Palmonari *et al.* were able to show that young people act in a selective way. Depending on the type of problem, reference may be made to parents, to peers or to both. Similar findings have been demonstrated in a Dutch study by Meeus (1989) and in a Scottish study by Hendry *et al.* (1993b).

Despite such selectivity much social cognitive research on adolescents has tended to concentrate on the content of young persons' thinking about people (O'Mahoney, 1986). Some attention has been given to how person-related constructs are applied (Jackson, 1987) but little attempt has been made to explore how social thinking develops and changes during adolescence, how it is modified by experience and how it is applied to the varied social worlds of adolescents.

Thus in addition to these fairly physical changes which herald the teenage years the adolescent has to achieve a variety of psycho-social tasks: Each adolescent must establish a sense of personal identity and self-esteem, must look for a personal philosophy and set of values, must aim for independence and adjust towards it. In addition, new relationships with adults and authority figures must be negotiated and roles clarified in respect of one's position with peers and with the opposite sex. At the same time external pressures force the young person to start adjusting towards an occupational (or unemployed/non-employed) role. Taken together these psycho-social factors interrelate to create and initiate the development of particular adult lifestyles.

Developing lifestyles

Coleman (1979) has presented a 'focal theory' arguing that the transition between childhood and adulthood cannot be achieved without substantial adjustments of both a psychological and social nature. Nevertheless, despite the amount of overall change experienced, most young people are extremely resilient and appear to cope with the necessary adjustments without undue stress.

Coleman's 'focal theory' offers a reason or rationale for this apparent contradiction. In it he proposed that at different ages particular sorts of relationship patterns come into focus at different times, but simply because an issue is not the most prominent feature at a particular age does not mean that it may not be critical for some individuals.

Coleman suggested that concern about gender roles and relationships with the opposite sex declines from a peak around 13 years; concerns about acceptance or rejection from peers are highly important around 15 years; while issues

15

regarding the gaining of independence from parents climb steadily to peak around 16 years and then begin to tail off. Such a theory may provide some insight into the amount of disruption and crisis implicit in adolesence and the relatively successful adaptation among most adolescents. The majority of teenagers cope by dealing with one issue at a time. Adaptation covers a number of years, with the adolescent attempting to solve one issue, then the next. Thus any stresses resulting from the need to adapt to new models of behaviour are rarely concentrated all at one time. Those who, for whatever reason, do have more than one issue to cope with at one time are most likely to have problems of adjustment:

> We believe that most young people pace themselves through the adolescent transition. Most of them hold back on one issue, while they are grappling with another. Most sense what they can and cannot cope with, and will, in the real sense of the term, be an active agent in their own development.
>
> (Coleman and Hendry, 1990, p.205)

The transitions of adolescence may be broadly similar for the majority of young people but the nature of the pathways followed through these transitions may vary widely according to a variety of psycho-social determinants and structural conditions. In order to take some account of these pathways and of the variability of development Hendry *et al.* (1993b) carried out a seven-year longitudinal study of young people growing up in the UK – the Young People's Leisure and Lifestyles Study (YPLL).

Hendry *et al.*'s lifestyle analysis (discussed in greater detail in Chapter 2) showed that lifestyles appeared to be clearly differentiated across a range of factors including health. These factors can be an interaction of self-perceptions, motivations, meanings and saliences which adolescents put upon various social and leisure activities; ecological influences such as socio-economic background; living conditions; parenting styles and family composition; school; peer groups and facets of wider cultural effects such as the mass media. These impinge on

16

social aspects of living in modern society such as being unemployed, moving on towards higher education or being
involved in risk-taking behaviours.

Risk behaviours

Though risk-taking has been one of the attributes of youth
since adolescence became recognized as a distinctive period of
the lifespan, the concept remains ill-defined. Are young people
at risk because they pursue different courses of action to
adults? Or do they pursue very similar courses of action but
are more vulnerable because they lack the learned ability to
resolve the situation to their advantage? From where does this
supposed predilection for risk-taking derive? Is it part of the
psychological make-up of youth – a thrill-seeking stage in a
developmental transition – a necessary rite of passage *en route*
to the acquisition of adult skills and self-esteem? Or is it a
consequence of a societal or cultural urge by adults to marginalize youth because their transition from controllable child to
controlled adult is a threat to the stability of the community?

In this 'at risk' scenario, young people as a population are
described as a 'problem' and the demands on education are
around socializing them more efficiently into the norms and
mores of adult society. As Hurrelman and Lösel (1990) have
suggested, personal behaviours in adolescence can contribute
to morbidity and mortality: smoking, heavy drinking, using
illegal drugs, precocious and unprotected sexual activity, no
regular participation in sports and exercise, traffic accidents,
violent, aggressive and delinquent activities 'indicate that the
image of "healthy adolescence" is inaccurate' (Hurrelmann
and Lösel, 1990, p.2).

Lewin (1970) argued that adolescents, in passing through
childhood to adulthood, are in a marginal position and entering a cognitively unstructured region. Their sense of
competence and ultimately their self-concept and future
personal identity depend on how well expectations are
accepted and processed into personal lifestyles at this stage of

17

development. If these behaviour patterns fit the requirements and rules encountered at school, at work, in relationships and in community life generally, then the outcome is satisfactory. Alternatively, if they fail to gain structure in their personal identity, confusion and conflict may result. Hence one cannot discount the possibility that crime and delinquency in our society are in some measure the cost of certain kinds of social development. It has been argued that the predominant ethic of our society is acquisitiveness and desire for success. But not everyone can be rich or successful legitimately. Several writers have pointed out that the values underlying juvenile delinquency may be far less deviant than is commonly assumed.

Some crimes reflect media images of the age and gender of the perpetrators. Much media attention has focused recently on the fad of joyriding – stealing cars and performing stunt tricks in them – even though relatively few young people are actually involved in this. More threateningly – as a recurring theme from the 1960s, the early and mid-1980s, and the early 1990s – several inner city areas of Britain witnessed events variously described as riots, disturbances and uprisings. The relationship between social deprivation, status frustration and race has moved juvenile crime to centre stage in policy matters:

> With the observation that there are gross differences in the rate of delinquency by class, by ethnic affiliation, by urban or rural residence, by region and perhaps by nation, from these gross differences the sociologist infers that something beyond the intimacy of family surroundings is operative in the emergence of delinquency patterns, something in the cultural and social atmosphere apparent in sections of society. (Wadsworth, 1979, p.3)

A number of qualifying points need to be made here: firstly, that the 'criminalizing' of certain forms of activity by adults may enhance their attraction and appeal for some young people, particularly if the activity is associated with media 'hype'; secondly, that labelling occurs when the same kind of activity is criminalized for some (e.g. soccer fans travelling to another town) and categorized as 'high spirits' in others

18

(e.g. misbehaviour on a rugby club outing). This labelling process also applies within the criminal system – often with a social class bias – in decisions about young people's appearance before children's panels or local magistrates and subsequent sentencing (Hendry and Shucksmith, 1994). Additionally, within the justice system young men and young women are often treated differently: young women are less likely to be brought to court, but if they are then they will be treated more harshly, and will be more likely to receive a custodial sentence.

Hence the adolescent years are a period when great adjustments have to be made by young people to changes both within themselves and in society and in relation to the expectations which society places on them. Many young people make the transition to adulthood with relative ease but some are handicapped by economic and structural forces which make their passage to a worthwhile adult status very difficult. Others have the misfortune to have to cope with too many challenges to their self-esteem and identity at one time. For some young people in these positions antisocial behaviour or self-destructive behaviour can be the consequence of their need to find either status or solace. Yet this deficit theory is not sufficient in itself to explain the attraction of taking risks, and it is important to have an understanding of the very positive attraction of thrilling and dangerous behaviours for some adolescents and the promises and denials held out to youth by the various sectors of adult society.

With regard to behaviours we need to ask why young people take risks. Firstly, there is a developmental factor. Many young people in their teenage years seek out thrills as earnestly as they did in childhood, perhaps to escape from a drab existence, to exert some control over their own lives, or to achieve something. Once we start to make the journey into adulthood there are fewer legitimate venues for thrill-seeking and the ones left open to us as adults often bear serious consequences. Those who see juvenile crimes only as a protest of the underprivileged deny the real thrill that such delinquent activities can inspire.

19

Over the past decade or so, Csikszentmihalyi and his colleagues at the University of Chicago have developed a model of optimal experience. It has also been called the flow model, 'flow' being the word used by interview subjects themselves to describe the experience of intense involvement in some activity – whether it be chess, rock climbing, dancing or performing heart surgery – where there is total concentration, little or no self-consciousness and a sense of self-transcendence resulting from a merging of consciousness with action (Csikszentmihalyi, 1975). The activities which afford such experience must be sufficiently challenging to engage a full measure of the individual's skill, but not so demanding as to be anxiety-provoking. Activities which provide clear feedback, such as those just mentioned, are most likely to be flow-producing. But the matching of challenges and skills is critical. If challenges are greater than skills, anxiety results, while a lack of challenge in relation to available skills is likely to be experienced as boredom. What is certain is that 'flow' in leisure provides a highly vivid climactic set of experiences. Descriptions of the feeling of flow indicate an experience that is totally satisfying beyond a sense of having fun. Enjoyment of the feeling may be akin to a peak experience in quality but its value is considered to be in its promotion of psychological growth 'like a built-in thermostat that indicates whether we are operating at full capacity at the leading edge of growth' (Csikszentmihalyi and Larson, 1984, p.269). The experience of flow as promotive of psychological growth would seem particularly pertinent to the transitions of adolescence.

Massimini and Carli (1988) have shown that positive optimal experiences occur when the individual can exert personal control in activities (i.e. skills exceeding moderate challenge) rather than in 'flow' (i.e. high challenge matched by skills). Nevertheless much optimal experience – considered as high enjoyment – was reported in 'flow' situations. In addition, optimal experience in flow was characterized by high cognitive involvement. Adolescents who experienced 'flow' as optimal experience were found to have higher psychological well-being than those who did *not* experience 'flow' as highly enjoyable. What the 'flow' model does seem to suggest is that certain qualities intrinsic to a variety of leisure pursuits are conducive to mental well-being. Sport, for example, offers advantages in terms of structural conditions conducive to optimal experience, but it appears to fall short with respect to such things as self-expression and individuation (Kleiber and Rickards, 1985). Comparing it with other leisure activities, sport does not offer the intrigue and free interchange of certain casual peer involvements nor the sense of a personal tutorial to be found in one-to-one hobbies (for example, working on cars). Sport in general can be a very positive experience for certain adolescents, but as Csikszentmihalyi and Larson (1984) have pointed out, so too can socializing, eating and travelling in a car. So too, we could add, can stealing and driving away someone else's car, or injecting drugs as a form of 'flow' and control.

Thus, various leisure activities can (potentially) provide therapeutic effects and produce sound mental health. Yet little is known of the properties, contexts and motivations which generate emotional stability and positive effects for young people in present-day society. Young people who organize themselves for the purpose of playing games are well regarded for their potential to create developmentally important experiences in the process (Devereux, 1976). But games are certainly not the only medium around which children and adolescents will organize (nor are they particularly the best ones considering their vulnerability to being co-opted by the forces of organized sport). The possibility that illegal or deviant activities (for example, drug use) may be among the more attractive alternatives for youth should only be regarded as a challenge to the purpose of identifying and developing the wealth of abilities and interests which adolescents possess. Though the majority of young people are hard-working, law-abiding and conventional, some adolescents exhibit rebellion both in their self-presentation and in their behaviour. In relation to social problems in general a number of studies have emphasized the

21

role of identity processes in determining behaviour (Emler, 1984). The desire to identify with a peer group especially in mid-adolescence (Coleman and Hendry, 1990) requires adherence to particular types of behaviour and role performance which imposes a group conformity even when antisocial actions may result.

But it also appears that the quest for excitement and violence is symbolic in the sense that young people 'use' these behaviours to identify, however misguidedly, with adult patterns of behaviour. Research has focused, especially, on drug and alcohol use, cigarette smoking, sexual behaviour and delinquency (Jessor and Jessor, 1977). Most of these behaviours would not be alarming if seen in adults but are perceived as being inappropriate for young people in the process of growing up. Silbereisen *et al.* (1987) have proposed that a number of so-called antisocial activities are in fact purposive, self-regulating and aimed at coping with aspects of adolescent development. They can play a constructive developmental role at least over a short term. Early sexual activity and early childbearing may have similar functions in providing a positive role and goal in young people's lives (Petersen *et al.*, 1987). While such behaviour is symbolic (i.e. these activities are usually engaged in because of a desire to create a self-image of maturity or as a perceived means of attaining attractiveness and sociability) they nevertheless can put adolescents at risk. Like adults, teenagers typically adopt behaviours in the belief that they will help achieve some desired end such as giving pleasure or gaining peer acceptance. In doing so they are likely to ignore or discount evidence that particular behaviours may pose potential threats to them. For example, a willingness to start smoking can be affected by beliefs adolescents hold about peer expectations and practices. In such instances a behaviour such as smoking may serve a wide range of purposes from projecting a desired image to emulating or defying an important authority figure.

Many of the explanations regarding adolescent risk behaviour thus rest on accounts of the development of the individual. Both Irwin (1989) and Jack (1989), for instance, consider that risk-taking is a normal transitional behaviour during adolescence. Indeed risk-taking is seen as fulfilling developmental needs related to autonomy and the need for mastery and individuation (Irwin and Millstein, 1986). In practice, what those who work with young people observe is a perceived invulnerability (or as Plant and Plant, 1992, would have it, an imagined invulnerability) to danger, whether this is in relation to road traffic accidents, or to the consequences of overindulgence in alcohol, smoking and so on. Elkind (1985) has characterized this as the 'Personal Fable' and has described its role in assuring adolescents that they are special and unique. In other words, it allows young people to enhance their self-esteem by believing that they can perform risky acts without experiencing the negative sequelae.

Children and young people like the rest of us experience inequality according to social class, gender, ethnicity and disability but their experience cannot be fully understood unless the lack of empowerment associated with their age is also recognized (Frost and Stein, 1989). This inability to view things from young people's perspective often provokes their alienation from adult society. There should be growing concern in society about the powerlessness of youth and its impact on their health and welfare in situations such as home-lessness or unemployment. At the same time, adult society *is* concerned with young people's apparent alienation from the perceived traditional values of this society made visible by those (often a minority of teenagers) engaged in joyriding, under-age sexual relations, vandalism, 'breaking and entering', and drug abuse (Davis, 1990). Jessor (1991), however, points to the fact that many of the apparently organized patterns of adolescent risk behaviour stem from the social ecology of adolescent life rather than from purely psychological sources. Thus this ecology provides socially organized opportunities to learn risk behaviours together and normative expectations that they be performed together. Risk-taking, according to Jessor, is by definition, entwined with lifestyle. Hendry *et al.* (1993b) have used the results of a longitudinal and multifaceted study of adolescents to characterize youth lifestyles more explicitly and to relate them to health status and longer-term life chances. The results confirm other work emphasizing the connection between risk-taking and having an 'at-risk' status or being part of a vulnerable group. For young people already (often deeply) in trouble in other ways, the investment in safer non-risky behaviour hardly seems worth the extra effort.

The social factors that induce risk-taking in young people are characterized well by Bellaby (1990) in considering young motorcyclists. Young people, he states, are 'in a liminal state, caught in the transition between two relatively defined statuses'. He refers to the model developed by van Gennep (1960) to explain how primitive societies deal with such borderline groups, namely successive rituals of three types – separation, exclusion and incorporation. From people in this liminal state, currently separated and even excluded, we may expect experimentation with new 'styles of life', venturing beyond the conventional and taking risks. Cultural theory would have it, that, having thus excluded our young adults and thus provoked their risk-taking behaviour, we are also likely to use their status of being 'at risk' or vulnerable to try to control or police their actions. It is important, therefore, to examine not only how differently risk-taking is perceived by young people and by their elders, but also to explore how those elders seek to contain risk-taking behaviour through societal restraints or through institutional forms. Such ambivalence is important to acknowledge and it raises many questions about the practices of all the professional groups and agencies working with young people in a rapidly changing society.

2 Young people's health

Introduction

We noted at the start of Chapter 1 how much attention is given in the media to aspects of youth culture seemingly opposed to traditional lifestyles and values. This vision of the opposition of youth may be overstated. Parental values and norms seem to be transmitted fairly steadily across the generation gap despite the separation in appearance, fashion and leisure activities bolstered by commercial interests (Coleman and Hendry, 1990). Since young people are reared in a social milieu which is quite different from that of their parents, individuals have to 'carry' with them into society the stamp of their own particular family lifestyle, yet tailored to suit young people's contemporary social requirements. In this way the rules and values of adolescent groups are influenced and altered, although most adolescents create lifestyles that are fairly consistent with their sub-cultural heritage. During adolescence young people are exposed to new social situations and need different social skills than those required in earlier childhood (Grinder, 1978). The shift from childhood to adolescence is marked by change in many aspects of social life (Damon, 1983). During adolescence peer relations become more intense and extensive, family relations are altered, and the adolescent begins to encounter many new demands, expectations and social contexts. Adolescents may begin dating, working with others in a part-time job, or spending time with their peers without adult supervision. Several developmental changes serve to alter the manner in which adolescents

25

interact with others. These include more advanced cognitive, verbal and reasoning abilities and the changes associated with puberty.

In considering the picture as a whole there seems little doubt that some of the most important events to which young people have to adjust are the multitude of physiological and bodily changes which occur during early adolescence and which are associated with what is generally known as puberty. Because of the complexities of modern society young people now approach physical maturity before many of them are capable of functioning well in adult social roles. The disjunction between physical capabilities, socially approved independence and power and the ambiguities in their current status can be stressful for some young people. Extreme examples of this increasing concern about 'body image', refusal to 'grow up', or 'rejection of an adult body shape', often reinforced by 'desirable' adult stereotypes and role models can set an adolescent on the pathway to anorexia or bulimia (Boskind-White and White, 1987). A publication aimed at young people (*Young Scot*, 1993) pointed out that in a study of 4,000 young people in Scotland, 40 per cent of 15-year-olds said they thought they should lose weight, half were already on some sort of diet, while separate figures showed that 1 per cent of adolescent British girls are now anorexic.

The transition to adulthood contains within it, the 'taking on' of adult-like behaviours with associated health concerns. Our knowledge of such patterns of young people's health understanding, behaviours and development comes from a variety of different types of research carried out with adolescent populations. Some of these are methodologically flawed, and we begin by examining this problem, since it affects the validity of what we *think* we know about young people's health and establishes the argument that more collaborative approaches with young people might enhance both the reliability and validity of our work. The chapter then goes on to select a number of health topics around each of which a discussion is based as to what we know of young people's behaviour, concerns and activities. In doing this we are inevitably falling into the trap identified by us elsewhere, namely, of problematizing youth health and of organizing our discussion around issues which give concern to adults rather than necessarily to young people themselves.

We aim to redress this balance somewhat towards the end of the chapter by the inclusion of a number of accounts derived from more qualitative or ethnographic-type studies. These have the virtue not only of demonstrating an alternative methodological framework for research on young people's health, but also of offering young people's accounts and agendas in a contextualized way.

Some methodological issues

Much of the current information on health habits like smoking and drinking has been gathered by means of large-scale representative surveys using self-completion questionnaires. This raises questions about the validity or truthfulness of some of the information volunteered by young people. Individuals may have reasons either for exaggerating behaviours which (to them) seem admirable, or for concealing behaviours which may be illegal or strongly condemned by society generally or the peer group in particular. Belief in the confidentiality of such research methods is often far from absolute. Additionally, these surveys are usually planned and implemented from an adultist – rather than from a young person's – perspective.

Further caveats have to be issued with regard to the comparability of surveys. The form of question will clearly influence the type of response given and too little attention is paid to this fact in the reporting of many surveys. Then, too, it is difficult to interpret the definitional boundaries or categories in some studies. 'Heavy smokers', for example, may be differently defined in studies, making comparability difficult.

Such survey data serve a purpose in keying us into general trends, but it is really in the *disaggregation* of the figures that facts of real importance emerge. Which is more interesting as a fact – that 18 per cent of all 15-year-olds smoke, or that significantly more girls than boys smoke at this age, that smoking peaks at 15 to 16 and thereafter declines, or that youngsters in certain socio-economic groups are more likely to smoke? Certainly, in targeting health promotion or evaluating where field interventions might be focused it is the disaggregated figures that are more illuminating. Methodological problems raise their head, however, in attempting to pursue this to its logical conclusion. Even large-scale nationally representative surveys have difficulty in producing results down to the local level (for instance, of a school catchment or neighbourhood) and illustrating differences which are statistically significant, simply because of the small cell sizes at these levels. Some health behaviours, notably those related to illicit drug use or sexual activity are difficult to handle sensitively within the format of a self-completion questionnaire or even a face-to-face interviewer completion survey. This is true of any age group, but is particularly pertinent in dealing with younger adolescents where parental or school consent may be withdrawn if questions are deemed to promote, imply or normalize 'deviant' health behaviours in any way.

In such circumstances qualitative research methods may be a more appropriate approach (and we will look at some of these studies later in this chapter). Such methods rely on direct interviewing of respondents, participant observation of activities, behaviours and lifestyles, the keeping of diaries and so on. Typically, however, such studies, because of their intensive nature, are small in size and are rarely able to boast a sample which is statistically representative. Nevertheless, their value is both in providing illuminative insights into the aggregated figures offered by quantitative surveys, and in triangulating and thereby validating information on health behaviours collected elsewhere.

Despite these problems in methodology a range of studies in the UK offer us useful information concerning the state of young people's health in Britain and highlight a variety of youth health issues.

Diet, nutrition and exercise

Whatever the discrepancies in the welfare state of the 1990s no adolescents are likely to starve in Britain. One of our concerns in relation to diet and nutrition rests in the type and quality of the food that young people consume. Are particular sections of the community further disadvantaged by the nature of their food intake in terms of day-to-day behaviour and short-term academic performance and long-term health? For instance, malnutrition among the young homeless may be more widespread than expected (Bridges Project, 1988). An additional concern relates to obsessive patterns of eating which often emerge in adolescence.

Complex studies of the dietary habits of the adult population demonstrate a change in eating trends. Older respondents to such surveys are more likely to eat three meals a day and to have breakfast. Whichelow (1987) reported that in the youngest age group surveyed (18 to 39 years) over one-third of respondents did not eat breakfast. The most striking difference was found between smokers and non-smokers, however. Smokers were far less likely to eat breakfast despite the fact that they were concentrated in manual occupations where physical effort was involved in their work.

The variations in diet by socio-economic class are well known. People in unskilled or semi-skilled occupations are likely to eat less fruit and vegetables, less brown bread and fewer wholemeal products, less meat and more fatty foods like chips. Gender differences are also worth noting, women on the whole eating more fruit, vegetables and salads, more low fat spreads and so on. Although there are regional differences in food consumption and eating patterns these are relatively small compared to socio-economic, age and gender differences.

The Mayfly study (Balding, 1986) looked in some detail at the nutritional intake of a non-representative sample of school children, but pointed out the 'fragile' nature of much of the information. Even when diaries were kept by respondents,

29

quantities were vague (one sandwich, a helping of potatoes) and the methods of preparation unknown. This study was particularly concerned with passing information back to schools to give them an indication of how well nourished their pupils were, so the vast array of data on this subject was re-coded on to a scale based on assumptions about the needs of pupils. The conclusion was that anyone scoring in the three lower categories was having a 'less than adequate' diet at some point in the day, and schools were concerned at finding a considerable percentage of pupils in this group. When food quantities were averaged out over the day 2 per cent of boys and 3 per cent of girls were 'starvers', on a minimal diet of only one drink or a single food item at each meal. Twenty-two per cent of boys and 27 per cent of girls were in categories 0 to 2 (demonstrating an existence based on 'snack' items). In terms of the quality and balance of diets, 48 per cent of boys and 39 per cent of girls had a diet assessed as being nutritionally deficient. Over half the girls in this study (57 per cent) reported having tried to exert some control over their weight, but only 20 per cent of the boys declared having done so.

A study carried out in Strathclyde (MacIntyre *et al.*, 1989) is more difficult to use for comparison because of the different nature of the data collection, but some interesting points emerge. While the majority of schoolchildren in that study either went home for lunch or had school meals in one form or another, 14 per cent of young people were going to 'take-aways' or cafés for this meal. Apart from these lunch-time visits, 36 per cent of young people had at least one other meal a week from a take-away, with 10 per cent of the sample having two or three evening meals a week from this source.

Physical activity

Another aspect of adolescent lifestyles which concerns adult society is young people's involvement in physical activity and sport. This is (at least partly) because of the high incidence of cardiovascular disease in the adult population generally and a desire to inculcate active lifestyles to counter this in the young. This has led to an intensive promotion of leisure sports, dominated by the notion of 'Sport for All' (European Sports Charter, 1975).

A number of research studies in the UK offer us some indications about young people's involvement in exercise and physical activity. Indeed Nichols and Mahoney (1989) have designed a test battery for the assessment of school-based cardiovascular fitness exercise potential. The work of Almond (1983) has demonstrated that English schoolchildren are involved in limited daily activity and certainly in little that increases their cardiovascular response. Nevertheless the studies of Balding (1986), Currie *et al.* (1987), MacIntyre *et al.* (1989) and Hendry *et al.* (1989) all indicate a high involvement of school-age children in fairly regular physical activity. Why then the apparent contradiction between Almond's work and other studies in this field? The answer lies in the fact that Almond's approach was particularly concerned with cardiovascular response while the others were looking at a wider involvement of young people in activity and not simply in structured school-based physical activities.

The Young People's Leisure and Lifestyle project (Hendry *et al.*, 1993b) has shown that among school pupils there is a relatively high involvement in physical activities, but differences obtain in relation to age and gender. Put simply, younger adolescents and male adolescents are most likely to be involved in physical activities and sports. There is a 'drop off' in involvement in the last few years of secondary schooling and particularly when young people make the transition from school towards work, training or higher education. Beyond the school years the social class position of young people derived from their occupational status produces clear differences in health and fitness levels.

We can draw together a number of important points from a range of research studies related to young people's involvement in physical activity. Firstly, organized sports and physical activities are not particularly attractive to certain adolescent

31

groups (e.g. young women), nor at certain times in the adolescent tradition (e.g. mid-adolescence and leaving school). Secondly, interest or relative disinterest in exercise and activity may be related to general attitudes towards school and schooling. Thirdly, despite the drop-off in involvement in organized activities, casual fun-oriented physical activities can be popular with young people, and particularly with young women when there is more focus on sociability, enjoyment and competence rather than a focus on competition. Fourthly, there is a need for intervention and research to examine the importance of motivation, context and values in relation to young people's involvement in activity and exercise. Fifthly, it is important to consider the salient elements within activity and exercise that would attract young people to continue involvement. Long-term goals associated with cardiovascular health do not seem to be sufficiently potent as an impetus for young people's participation. Finally, we need to be aware of the possibly 'competing' leisure and social activities that young people may be involved in and to be alert to Balding's (1987) comments about the effects of the mass media in projecting 'desirable' adult social stereotypes. This can often prevent young people perceiving physical activity and exercise as being a necessary and valuable part of adult lifestyle. For example, Hendry and Singer (1981) found that a sample of adolescent girls had very positive *attitudes* towards physical activity for health reasons but assigned low priority to their actual involvement in these pursuits because of 'conflicting' interests and saliences – usually of a social nature, related to visiting friends, going to discos and 'courting'.

Smoking

Golding (1987) has noted that the decrease in smoking in industrialized countries has been dramatic. In three decades, smoking prevalence among adult United Kingdom males has fallen from 70 per cent to 40 per cent, for example. However, within this general trend a number of themes in relation to gender, social class and age gradients in smoking prevalence can be noted. Among Golding's adult population, 'current regular cigarette smoking' rates (a respondent currently smoking more than one cigarette per day) were at 35 per cent of men and 31 per cent of women. However, 44 per cent of the youngest male cohort (18 to 20 years) had 'never smoked'. Strong socio-economic group gradients were noted in the adult population, the prevalence of smoking being highest in the 'unskilled manual' and lowest in the 'professional' groups. Regional differences also existed, with smoking prevalence being higher in northern England and Scotland. How far are these characteristics replicated in the adolescent population?

The Social Survey Division of the Office of Population Censuses and Surveys (OPCS) carried out a series of studies of smoking among secondary school children in the 1980s. A number of problems emerge in looking at this data, not least of which is the fact that 'regular' smoking is defined as smoking at least one cigarette a week, a category threshold so low as to be intuitively rather worrying. From these figures, however, it appears that among the adolescent population the prevalence of 'regular' smoking has indeed declined. The 1986 OPCS figures show rates in Scotland being higher and a bigger difference appearing between the rates for boys and girls, with girls being more likely to smoke than boys. Among those who do smoke, boys continue to be heavier smokers than girls. A study of school pupils aged 14 to 15 carried out in the 1980s on a non-representative sample, for instance, found that the average daily consumption of girl smokers was six cigarettes, compared with eight cigarettes for boys (Balding, 1986). Balding speculates that at least part of the explanation for this discrepancy might lie in the earlier social maturity of girls. In other words, the fact that girls tend to socialize with boys who are older than themselves might make it more logical to compare the smoking of 15-year-old girls with that of 17-year-old boys, for example. Goddard (1989) in a study of schoolchildren found that adolescents were much more likely to be smokers if other people at home smoked. Brothers and sisters appeared to have more influence in this respect than did parents. These results are confirmed in a study of Scottish adolescents undertaken by the present authors (Glendinning *et al.*, 1992).

Coggans *et al.* (1990) undertook a large-scale prevalence study as part of a national evaluation of drug education. The young people in this study were all in the second, third or fourth year of their secondary school careers and were identified as representative of the range both of social class and drug education experience typifying Scottish school pupils in these age groups though the pupil sample was drawn entirely from the Central Belt of Scotland. Something like 15 per cent of the Coggans sample smoked at the 'regular' level (defined by OPCS as at least one cigarette a week). Such a figure may seem to reverse the trend of decline in smoking in this age group, but the rise is likely to be a consequence of differences in sampling procedure. Davies and Coggans (1991) noted the strangely bimodal distribution of smoking in the adolescent population, one sizable group smoking very infrequently (19 per cent), and the other group (14 per cent) being frequent smokers. Trends within this dataset replicate those in the OPCS studies. In other words, older adolescents are more likely to smoke than younger ones, females are more likely to smoke than males and young people from lower socio-economic groups are more likely to smoke than their counterparts in higher socio-economic groups.

Data collected in 1987 on a 15-year-old cohort by MacIntyre *et al.* (1989) confirmed the trends noted above. Just over 12 per cent of 15-year-olds in this regional sample claimed to smoke regularly (quantities were not defined), but the rate varied from 10 per cent in middle-class districts to 19 per cent in a principally working-class area, highlighting the social class differences noted above. Further evidence on the link with social class comes from the Young People's Leisure and Lifestyle study (Hendry *et al.*, 1993b), in which 19 per cent of 13- to 24-year-olds considered themselves to be smokers. Overall in the data a clear trend with age is discernible, with the proportion of smokers rising to a peak in the early twenties and then falling slightly.

Of most interest, however, is the fact that social class differences, when measured in the traditional way by social class of head of household were non-significant though the trend was in the same direction noted in other studies ('non-manual' adolescents providing 11 per cent of regular smokers, and those from a manual background providing 14 per cent of regular smokers). However, for the oldest four cohorts it was possible to measure *current* social class rather than class of origin. In other words, the current socio-economic position occupied by young people themselves at the time of the survey was measured (e.g. in full-time education, employed in semi-skilled occupation etc.) Using this measure, significant differences do emerge in smoking status between groups of young people engaged in different types of economic activity. For example, only 11 to 13 per cent of young people in further education or professional and intermediate categories were 'regular' smokers, compared with 28 per cent of the unemployed.

Alcohol

Measuring consumption of alcohol poses as many problems as measuring smoking prevalence. Studies requiring respondents to classify themselves as 'light' or 'heavy' drinkers can produce very variable results – one person's 'light' may be another person's 'heavy'! One of the best methods of validating the data is by comparison of diaries of drinking. Specific information on what has been drunk as well as the quantity can enable the researcher to convert the declared consumption into units of pure alcohol and apply definitions of light, moderate and heavy with more precision. These definitions also apply different standards to men and women, a customary practice justified not only by typical differences in body weight and in social norms but also by the evidence that the threshold where consumption becomes damaging in women may be lower than in men. Overall there is a problem of under-reportage of drinking levels, though the reverse may be true in adolescent populations, and this is particularly likely in surveys of a more general kind. In surveys focused specifically on alcohol consumption interviewers may be more skilled at eliciting reliable information.

Among the adult population (Blaxter, 1987) there are big regional differences in drinking pattern and alcohol consumption, with the heaviest consumers among men being in the north of England, Scotland and Wales, and the heaviest consumers among females being in Yorkshire, Greater London and the West Midlands. Blaxter commented that the social characteristic most regularly associated with greater consumption is income. This results in a patterns of heavier drinking among men in managerial, self-employed manual and skilled manual occupational classes at younger ages, and in professional, employers and managers classes in middle age. The retired and the unemployed drink less. Women who work outside the house drink more than housewives. Divorced/separated men and women are particularly likely to be moderate or heavy drinkers. Among adults the pattern of their own parents' drinking is a powerful determinant of their own drinking status. Women's drinking is particularly clearly associated with that of their mothers.

Are these patterns reproduced in the adolescent population? The literature on young people drinking describes such behaviour as part of the socialization process from child to adult (Stacey and Davies, 1970; Barnes, 1977; Sharp and Lowe, 1989). In England and Wales, the majority of adolescents have had their first 'proper' drink by the age of 13 (82 per cent of boys, and 77 per cent of girls). In Scotland, schoolchildren are introduced to alcohol a little later (71 per cent of 12-year-old boys and 57 per cent of girls) but catch up with their English and Welsh peers by the age of 15 (Marsh *et al.*, 1986). Lest these young drinkers cause great concern, it needs to be pointed out that most only drank alcohol a few times a year. Most adolescents' early drinking is done at home with parents.

Only as they grow older does the context for their drinking spread to parties, then clubs and discos and lastly to pubs. Scottish adolescents are much less likely than their English and Welsh counterparts to drink in pubs. Marsh *et al.* (1986) comment:

> Among the younger Scottish adolescents, particularly the 14 and 15 year olds, the proportion who claim usually to drink in pubs is small, less than half the values claimed in England and Wales. Scottish adolescents are far more likely to say they drink 'elsewhere'. Since this is not at home, nor on licenced premises, 'elsewhere' must be mostly outside on the streets, or wherever else Scottish adolescents may drink unobserved by parents or authorities.   (Marsh *et al.*, 1986, p.19)

Most young people's drinking is done at weekends, as diary evidence shows. In relation to quantities, girls in every age group drank less than boys in the OPCS (1986) survey. Boys' consumption grows annually, with some very high levels being reached by age 17, whereas girls' consumption peaks in the last year of schooling. In Scotland, boys on average drink three times more than girls.

Data from the YPLL survey confirm the trends noted above, with 5 per cent of 13- to 14-year-olds being 'frequent drinkers' (once a week or more often), rising to 48 per cent of 17- to 18-year-olds and 66 per cent of 23- to 24-year-olds (which would obviously include students). In this sample of 65 per cent of 17- to 18-year-olds went to a pub once a month or more. Pub-going seemed to peak in the late teens and thereafter tail off.

No significant differences emerged in drinking behaviour over the whole sample in terms of gender although, in the youngest two cohorts, boys were more likely to be frequent drinkers and to be buying alcohol from supermarkets. Across the whole sample there were no significant differences in drinking prevalence by social class of head of household. An analysis of the drinking data for the oldest four cohorts by a residential neighbourhood classification (i.e. ACORN Classification: Shaw, 1984) showed raised levels of frequent

37

drinking in the most affluent areas, but this was not statistically significant. Analysis by school catchment of the youngest groups of children did, however, show significant variability. The Highlands and Islands catchments showed the smallest proportion of youngsters who never drank. Two of these three catchments also held the highest proportions of frequent drinkers (approximately 16 per cent of those who drank). The proportion of frequent drinkers ranged between 2 per cent and 18 per cent, indicating the variety of local 'cultures' within which young people drink.

While the long-term health consequences of regularly drinking large amounts of alcohol are well understood, there are also short-term health and social consequences of infrequent but very heavy drinking. Consequently some of the data on 'drunkenness' is actually of more interest. In the OPCS survey (Marsh *et al.*, 1986) about 30 per cent of the youngest boys and 23 per cent of the youngest girls who drank in Scotland admitted to being 'very drunk' once or more than once. It is important to note that these figures do not include young people who were not drinkers. Bearing in mind the caveat that such measurements are very subjective, it would seem that such behaviour peaks for both boys and girls at age 15, but declines more rapidly for girls thereafter.

The majority of adolescents associate drinking with positive reactions, but Marsh *et al.* (1986) noted that associated with such specific bouts of drunkenness were not only the inevitable physical symptoms but also drinking-related problems such as vandalism, attracting the attention of the police and so on. The findings suggest that

> for a minority of adolescents, probably a small minority, drinking to excess is an established habit. (Marsh *et al.*, 1986)

Coffield (1992) in a more up-to-date study of young people in the north-east of England makes the following comment:

> The pattern of weekend 'binges' appears to be widespread among both young men and young women and underage drinking seems to be endemic throughout the region. As a result of drinking too

much, boys become involved in fights among themselves, with other male groups and with the police; they also damaged themselves and others in accidents with motorbikes and cars; their relationships with parents became strained, and some became more willing to experiment with illicit drugs after drinking heavily. If any of the girls became involved with the police, it was in connection with drink-related offences. Among the young people we met, the non-drinker is the deviant and talk of sensible drinking is openly ridiculed. Our young people reported very few hangovers, although they were often sick as a result of excessive drinking. They tend to dismiss any possible health risks because they 'bounce back' so quickly and without any apparent ill-effects. They find it difficult, if not impossible, at the age of 15 'to worry about the health of a 50 year old stranger i.e. themselves 35 years in the future'. (Coffield, 1992, pp.2–3)

Drugs

In introducing their audit of drug misuse statistics, the authors of a report published by the Institute for the Study of Drug Dependence (Ashton, 1991) points out that whereas for alcohol, tobacco and prescribed medicines, good national statistics are readily to hand, beyond these socially 'approved' forms of drug use, statistical provision is patchy and of little direct relevance to the issue of how many people misuse drugs.

This problem will dog us in describing patterns of drug use, though in some senses the diversity of small-scale studies on this topic highlights the localized nature of many cultures of drug misuse and points more clearly to ways and means of intervention at local levels than do uniform or national statistics.

One of the forms of drug misuse associated with the youngest adolescent is solvent misuse. Misuse of solvents is discouraged both because of the short-term and long-term dangers to health and safety that they present. One of the characteristic features of solvent misuse is that it is often very localized and very transitory, becoming wildly popular with a cohort of young people on a particular estate or in a school, for instance, then quickly disappearing. So, in some places at some times, large numbers of children will be experimenting, but only a few of these young people will carry on misusing solvents after the 'fad' has passed. British studies (Ives, 1990a) suggest that between 4 per cent and 8 per cent of secondary school pupils have tried solvents, and that sniffing peaks around ages 13 to 15 (third and fourth year of secondary schooling in England, second and third year of schooling in Scotland). In Davies and Coggans' sample, nearly 11 per cent of the sample had used solvents at least once although less than 1 per cent reported using solvents once a month or more frequently. Most of those who had used solvents had used them only once or a few times (Davies and Coggans, 1991).

However, despite the low incidence of continued misuse, it is clear that the fashion for solvent misuse has not gone away despite attracting less media attention in recent years. Numbers of solvent-related deaths give some indication of the problem's continuation. In 1983, when concern was at its highest, deaths totalled 82. In 1988 there were 134 deaths, more deaths per annum than are attributed to the misuse of any other illegal drug in the adolescent population (Wright, 1991). Part of the concern rests in the fact that published guidelines to retailers on the sale of glues – the most well-known solvent – have led to a trend towards misuse of more dangerous products such as aerosols (Ives, 1990b; Ramsey, 1990).

More common in usage among adolescents is cannabis, ranking third behind alcohol and cigarettes as a preferred drug. Davies and Coggans (1991) note that although 15 per cent of their sample of school-age children had tried cannabis at least once, only 2 per cent carried on using it about once a month or more frequently.

Cannabis is not in itself addictive and, although linked with short-term memory problems and other minor symptoms, is not associated with any significant long-term damage to health. It is, however, an illegal substance, and thus most of the problems associated with its use stem from social rather than medical causes. There is some evidence that young people view cannabis in quite a different light from those offering health education on the topic (Hendry *et al.*, 1991b). Those concerned with health promotion for young people are often bound by professional guidelines to group cannabis with other illegal drugs and must effectively prohibit its use. Young people's own culture, however, denies that cannabis is harmful – it is often seen as less dangerous than alcohol, both in terms of the quantities consumed and the fact that it is less likely than alcohol to provoke violent behaviour. The association of cannabis with other illegal substances diminishes the validity of the message that health educators promote. The study reported by Davies and Coggans (1991) demonstrates how low is the incidence of other illegal drugs in school-age populations. Six per cent reported having used LSD at least once. Figures for heroin and cocaine were 1 per cent. Ecstasy was recorded at below 1 per cent of young people having used it, although more recent surveys might highlight the fashion in use of such designer drugs in dance settings. Informal sources, however, indicate that the use of Ecstasy ('E') is actually in decline after an initial burst of enthusiasm for the drug, for reasons of cost and impurity. Amphetamines or 'speed' have, however, replaced 'E' as a popular choice with young people, at least in the Edinburgh area (Fast Forward, 1994).

However, Davies and Coggans comment:

> Data of this sort are reassuring for parents worried about the probability of their children taking drugs, but it should be said that this low level of probability is not evenly spread throughout society.
>
> (Davies and Coggans, 1991, p.36)

No direct question was asked about personal drug-taking behaviours in the YPLL study (Hendry *et al.*, 1993b) but young people were asked both about their attitudes to drug-taking and about the proportions of young people in their peer group who used drugs. Boys were more likely than girls to state that some of their close friends used drugs. Age 17 to 18 was the peak period for drug use with 41 per cent of this age group claiming that some of their close friends used drugs.

There was a significant link between those claiming a close friend as a drug user and social class, with 32 per cent of young people from professional or intermediate social classes making this claim compared to 23 per cent of those from semi-skilled or unskilled social classes. One could postulate that this puts the lie to theories about use of drugs in general and social deprivation, and highlights the advent of expensive designer drugs or the predominance of cannabis. This was reinforced by analysing those claiming to have close friends who used drugs by the ACORN variable – the measure of residential neighbourhood type. Significant differences emerged, with the lowest declarations of drug use among peers in agricultural areas (16 per cent) and the highest (48 per cent) in affluent areas of private housing. Of particular interest from this study are the data on this topic for the oldest cohorts analysed by the current social class of the respondents themselves. The results demonstrate a distinctly bimodal distribution in which the highest claims for drug use among friends are in the groups currently engaged in higher education and those who are unemployed.

Sex and sexuality

Adolescent sexual behaviour has always been a cause of concern to adults in society. Fears about sexual activity leading to unwanted pregnancy are coupled with a desire to protect the younger adolescent from exploitation and pressure to become sexually active before they have the emotional or social maturity to cope. Apart from risks to mental and social well-being, there are risks to health both in the short term and long term. Early pregnancies are associated with increased risk for both mother and baby; early onset of sexual behaviour has been statistically linked in females with cancers of the reproductive organs appearing in later life, and sexually transmitted diseases pose threats to the health and well-being of young people of both sexes.

In recent years, of course, the spread of HIV through sexual activity has caused increased focus to be put on young people's activities. Bury comments:

> Teenagers are often regarded as key factors in the future of the heterosexual epidemic. Unfortunately this is sometimes due to myths about their sexual behaviour, as they are often seen as promiscuous and irresponsible in their attitude to protection. Although there is much evidence to suggest that this image misrepresents the vast majority of teenagers in Britain, teenagers do remain a key factor in the heterosexual epidemic for other reasons. Adolescence is a time of experimentation; young people tend to see themselves as invulnerable, yet they are particularly vulnerable when they are at the stage of seeking a sexual partner.
>
> (Bury, 1991, p.43)

The difficulties in obtaining accurate information either on sexual behaviours or on HIV status are almost too well known to need rehearsing. Recent figures for Scotland attesting to the fact that 9 per cent of those infected with HIV (i.e. 8 per cent of infected men and 12 per cent of infected women) are aged between 15 and 19, highlight, however, the need to know about the reality of young people's sexual behaviour and attitudes so that appropriately targeted health interventions can be made. There have been two main studies of young people's sexual behaviour in Britain, one in the mid-1960s (Schofield, 1965) and the other ten years later (Farrell, 1978). Since then all other studies have been localized and small scale, apart from Johnson *et al.*'s (1994) recent research which included questions concerning age of first intercourse, sexual experience and lifestyles.

Earlier Ford (1987) identified the important indicators of patterns of heterosexual activity as age at first intercourse, the level of premarital sex, the number of sex partners and the proportion using a condom. With regard to the first of these, the trend has been for teenagers to begin sexual intercourse at a younger age than in the past (e.g. Farrell, 1978; Ford and Bowie, 1989). Johnson *et al.* (1994) have shown that the age for first heterosexual intercourse reveals a pattern of decreasing age at occurrence, together with an increase in the proportions reporting sexual experience before the age of 16, together with some convergence in the behaviour of young men and young women over time. In the past four decades the median age at first heterosexual intercourse has fallen from 21 to 17 years for women and from 20 to 17 years for men, while the proportion reporting its occurrence before the age of 16 has increased from fewer than 1 per cent of women now aged 55 years and over to nearly one in five of those now in their teens.

Social class differences in early sexual experience were significant in the 1970s, with young working-class men significantly more likely than their middle-class counterparts to be sexually experienced, but these differences appear to be less significant in more recent data collections (MORI, 1990; Wellings and Bradshaw, 1994; Wight, 1993). These changes need to be seen in the context of liberalizing legal reforms, advances in medical technology and changes in a permissive direction of social and sexual attitudes. The general impression seems to be one of increasing homogeneity with respect to gender, occupational and educational levels and other socio-demographic variables. Early intercourse is still associated with lower social class and low educational levels, but these effects are weakening. This is also true of 'current' social class (i.e. based on the young person's current level of economic activity rather than 'ascribed' social class (i.e. based on the occupation of the father). Ford and Bowie's (1989) work, for instance, suggests that those in full-time education are twice as likely not to have had sexual intercourse as those in full-time employment, housewives or the unemployed.

It is important to stress the vast diversity in the individual experiences of young people. Conger and Petersen (1984) make a particular point of emphasizing the importance of looking at individual differences when considering figures such as these. Apart from age, gender, socio-economic status and nationality, variables such as social class, ethnic origin and cultural background obviously play their part in determining sexual behaviour. The broad social trends described above also need to be considered in the light of other studies which have highlighted the different experience of young people in urban and rural settings (Johnson *et al.*, 1994). Ford and Bowie (1989) found only 56 per cent of youngsters in rural areas were sexually experienced compared with 70 per cent of their counterparts in urban and semi-urban areas.

Although teenagers are more likely to be sexually experienced than they have been in the past, there is no evidence that they are more likely to have casual sex relationships. Ford and Morgan (1989) claim that over 70 per cent of teenagers have intercourse only within a committed, loyal relationship. Bury (1984) and Wellings and Bradshaw (1994) have characterized adolescent sexual relationships as being 'serial monogamy'. Other studies seem to confirm this pattern (Abrams *et al.*, 1990). Such a claim would seem to be borne out by Stegen's (1983) and Tobin's (1985) studies of female teenage family planning clinic attenders. This evidence, now 10 years old, showed that approximately 90 per cent of those attending had had only one or two sexual partners, and they were clearly 'comfortable' with the social acceptance of their sexual activity.

Johnson *et al.* (1994) also report that first intercourse is now often associated with more planning and less spontaneity than formerly. They state that the majority of young people have their first experience of sexual intercourse within an established relationship. Young women are usually initiated by an older male partner, while young men's first partners tend to be age peers. It is uncommon, and increasingly so, for first intercourse to take place within marriage, and very rare for young men's first sexual intercourse to be with a prostitute.

A small proportion of young people have multiple sexual partners, and it is a behaviour possibly associated with emotional deprivation or serious psychological problems (Hein *et al.*, 1978). Studies which have focused on 'sexually delinquent' youth (those who have committed sexual offences against other persons) and runaways emphasize the very high-

45

risk pattern of sexual activity common in some groups which require very targeted and specific health education interventions (Rotherham-Borus *et al.*, 1991). Again there is a boundary problem as to how significant a problem this is seen to be. MORI (1990) reports that 11 per cent of 16- to 19-year-olds had four or more sexual partners in the previous year. Although some of these sexual encounters may have been monogamous and not undertaken in a promiscuous fashion at the time, there is clearly room for debate about the impact of such activities in increasing the risk factor for young people.

Contraceptive use among teenagers has risen in line with the rise in those claiming sexual experience in teenage years, but such use has been shown in numerous studies to be inconsistent. The condom is the only contraceptive which assists in the prevention of sexually transmitted diseases and the HIV virus. Bowie and Ford (1989) suggest that about a third of sexually active young people use condoms, but almost all claim to use them for contraceptive rather than disease prevention purposes (Hendry *et al.*, 1991). Despite the campaigning for condom use, a complex web of cultural and social factors conspire to make them unappealing and unusable for many young people, especially when other forms of contraception (e.g. the pill) are available (Wight, 1990). Despite the fact that contraception is difficult for many young people to access or negotiate with a partner, the evidence of data relating to teenage pregnancies attests to the fact that young women are no more likely now than in the past to conceive children at this early stage in their lives (Johnson *et al.*, 1994).

All of the foregoing relates to heterosexual activity. Very little is known about rates of homosexual activity among adolescents. Kent-Baguley (1990) notes that 'not surprisingly, the majority of young lesbians and gays feel marginalized, isolated and unhappy at school, often feeling obliged to participate in 'queer-bashing' talk to avoid self-revelation'. Little wonder that the extent of the phenomenon is so unclear. A MORI poll carried out for the Health Education Authority (MORI, 1990) asked 16- to 19-year-old respondents to place themselves on a scale indicating their sexual orientation. MORI concluded that 88 per cent in this age group were clearly heterosexual and only 1 per cent clearly homosexual. A further 6 per cent, however, were bisexual or had a bisexual orientation. Also in question is the extent to which homosexual practices place young people at risk. Blanket assumptions about the nature of sexual acts or the levels of promiscuity in this sub-group too often reflect simple stereotypes and prejudices. Young people themselves are particularly confused about the nature of the AIDS danger in relation to homosexuality since there is almost no discussion within health education about sexuality *per se* and homosexuality in particular.

Young people's lifestyles

Most of the work described in this chapter falls within the ambit of traditional epidemiological research. Aaro *et al.* (1986) describe the paradigm thus:

> In epidemiology it is important to identify statistical associations, to determine *causality* of relationships, and to quantify the strength of those relationships. Consequenctly, epidemiological research focuses strongly on those aspects of lifestyle and environment which it is possible to measure in mass surveys and which may have an impact on health. (Aaro *et al.*, 1986, p.18).

Research conducted within this paradigm allows us to establish national trends, to look at how trends change over time, to compare regions or sub-groups within the population. Often, it is impossible to disaggregate figures to the point where it would be possible to target health education or interventions very specifically or locally. Nor do such statistics tell us much about the social contexts within which specific behaviours take place. There is an oft-quoted gap between health knowledge and health behaviours in young people which remains puzzling and paradoxical if we stay within the traditional epidemiological mould. The puzzle may be resolved if the research is refocused within the lives and lifestyles of the

47

young people concerned, to look at the attitudes and reasons for actions.

Aaro *et al.* (1986) defined lifestyles as 'relatively stable patterns of behaviour, habits, attitudes and values which are typical for the groups one belongs to, or the groups one wants to belong to' (p. 19). Lifestyles are clearly developed through a process of socialization and encompass values and attitudes as well as actions. Lifestyle is clearly related, too, to socio-economic circumstances. The ease with which an individual may choose, change or adapt his or her lifestyle will depend on social situation, wealth and status. Abel and McQueen (1992) have put forward the idea that lifestyle consists of three dimensions, namely orientations, resources and behaviour. From this stance lifestyles are collective phenomena allowing for social differentiation within and between groups.

In looking at health through the focus of lifestyle a host of additional factors present themselves for consideration which would be of no concern in epidemiological research. An excellent example of this concerns young people's leisure time activities. The type and nature of interactions with parents and peers in leisure time is strongly associated with addictive behaviour like smoking or use of alcohol. Within a research model which focuses on lifestyle we must, then, look at a whole range of wider issues. Aaro *et al.* comment:

> Studying lifestyle from an epidemiological point of view may be compared to studying climate and weather processes from the periscope of a submarine. (Aaro *et al.*, 1986, p.19)

From an ecological perspective the groups a person belongs to are of vital importance. Young people belonging to a family with higher socio-economic status are exposed to different types of role models than working-class young people. This may also pertain to habits and behaviours associated with lifestyle patterns.

To summarize, our understanding of the development of adolescent lifestyles needs to take account of a 'network' of determinants and these include the individual with his or her socialization process and present personality as well as his or her immediate surroundings (family, teachers, friends, workmates and colleagues). It also includes connections within the social and economic environment. Thus objective conditions and subjective perceptions are contained within one model. In particular the linkages of this network help formulate a better understanding of the development of the constituent elements of lifestyles during adolescence.

The Young People's Leisure and Lifestyles project used cluster analysis to identify this network of linkages that go to make up lifestyles (Hendry *et al.* 1993b). Table 2.1 provides a brief description of types of adolescent lifestyle found. First, different lifestyles (clusters) are associated with different social class backgrounds. In fact, using parents' occupation, parents' level of education and the young person's local residential neighbourhood, it is possible to describe the clusters (lifestyles) nearer to the top of Table 2.1 as 'working-class' and those nearer to the bottom as 'middle-class'. These class labels are also consistent with the intended educational and employment trajectories of young people within the different clusters. For instance, among both young women and men, the middle-class clusters 4 and 5 are associated with the intention to go on to college or university before seeking employment.

Focusing on the results of the cluster analysis for young women and looking at the connections between health, sport and lifestyle, cluster 2 can be identified with an unhealthy lifestyle and cluster 4 with a healthy lifestyle. Young women in cluster 2 view themselves as less healthy and as more stressed and have little interest or involvement in sport, while young women in cluster 4 assess themselves as healthy and are involved in competitive sport and sports clubs. It would be a mistake to think of these two clusters as typical of the differences between a working-class lifestyle (cluster 2) and a middle-class lifestyle (cluster 4). If anything, young women in cluster 1 can be viewed as representative of a typically working-class lifestyle. They are health conscious, not subject

Table 2.1 *A typology of mid-adolescent lifestyle (15–16 years)*

Clusters for young women	Clusters for young men
1 (36%) From skilled, semi-skilled or unskilled classes; part-time job; health conscious; no stress; visited by and visit female friends often; gregarious; spend a lot of spare time with family; organized and casual leisure; play sport for recreation and go to sports fixtures	1 (7%) From semi-skilled classes; part-time job; won't continue education; view getting a job as a priority; content; hang about in street, but avoid trouble; disapprove of alcohol; feel parents are unsupportive; organized and casual leisure; think local sports facilities are poor, positive about sport, go to sports fixtures and play sport competitively
2 (6%) From skilled classes; dislike school; get a job rather than continue education, but not confident about finding one; less healthy and more stressed; not content; hang about in street; casual leisure only; bored; lots of spare time alone or with a best friend; little involvement in sport	2 (18%) From skilled, semi-skilled or unskilled classes; intend to get a job as soon as possible; feel stressed and view self as unfit; not outgoing; don't get on with father and parents unsupportive; little leisure; bored; little involvement in sport
3 (18%) From a mix of social backgrounds, but few from semi-skilled or unskilled classes; visited by and visit female friends often; more time with peers and a boyfriend and less time with family; family conflict; spend money on cigarettes; hang about in street; casual and commercial leisure; play sport for recreation	3 (16%) From skilled classes; part-time job; won't continue education; intend to enter manual employment and train on the job; not health conscious; outgoing; spend money on clothes; time with a girlfriend; don't disapprove of young people drinking; organized, casual and commercial leisure; hang about in street; play sport for recreation and go to sports fixtures

4 (7%) Professional, intermediate, skilled classes; intend to continue with education; confident about finding employment; healthy and content; disapprove of alcohol; spend a lot of spare time with family; get on with parents; or organized leisure; spend money on sports goods, member of a sports club and play competitive sport

4 (38%) Professional, intermediate, skilled classes; intend to continue with education and then enter non-manual employment; gregarious; health conscious; disapprove of alcohol; parents supportive and get on with them; organized leisure; buy sports goods, member of sports club and play competitive sport

5 (19%) Professional, intermediate, skilled classes; intend to continue with education; confident about finding employment; view self as healthy, but feel stressed; not content; little time with a close friend; little interest or involvement in sport.

5 (9%) Professional, intermediate, skilled classes; intend to continue with education and then enter non-manual employment; not content; disapprove of alcohol; spend much time alone; little organized or casual leisure; negative about sport, don't go to sports fixtures; little involvement in sport

(12%) Unclassified

(9%) Unclassified

(Source: Hendry *et al.*, 1993b)

to stress, have a network of female friends, get on well with their parents and regularly participate in sport, but for recreation only. The results also show there are distinctly different types of middle-class lifestyle. As has been shown, young women in cluster 4 can be regarded as having a healthy middle-class lifestyle. By contrast, although young women in cluster 5 are equally middle class and also assess themselves as healthy, they report significantly more stress and have little interest or involvement in sport.

Looking at the results for young men, broadly similar types of lifestyles are apparent and once again it is possible to connect these to health and sport. For example, young men in clusters 4 and 5 come from equally middle-class backgrounds, but males in the smaller cluster 5 tend to be unhappy, socially isolated and negative about sport, while those in the large cluster 4 are gregarious, health conscious and much involved in sport. Among working-class males, young men in the smaller cluster 1 are more involved in sport, while those in the larger cluster 2 have little interest in sport.

Ethnographic studies

Clearly, from the study described above, it is possible to research lifestyles using quantitative methods, yet it is in ethnographic type studies, that the richness and complexity of youth lifestyles is best revealed. A rich tapestry of data collected *in situ* has high validity. The people portrayed in such studies are real people and it is not difficult to picture their reactions to health education messages for example, or empathize with their problems in following good advice in the teeth of all the other social and economic pressures around them. Such studies are inevitably small scale. The danger, too, is that researchers are inevitably drawn to socially deviant behaviours or daring sub-groups. 'Ordinary' youngsters are a less attractive focus for such work, but predictably, the results from observation of such small and extraordinary groups are often extrapolated to form the basis for judgement on the majority. Thus it is useful to be able to balance the dramatic accounts of young people using drugs with statistics that point to how few people's lives are actually affected in this way.

The following three short examples of such work are presented to illustrate the style of this research, and to point to its value in explicating the nature of the competing claims on young people in social situations which makes health choices so difficult. In this way it is hoped that the value of such work in identifying realistic community interventions will be recognized.

Drink and 'the new lawlessness'

The emergence of the 'lager lout' in recent years has generated considerable media attention. Young drinkers are blamed for innumerable instances of disorderliness in county towns or on football terraces. Tragedies such as those at the Hysel stadium or Hillsborough are blamed on drunkenness. What seems to generate most distress in the tabloid newspapers is that these are patently not young people without hope, drinking to relieve their sorrows. Many of the young people involved have good jobs and reasonable incomes. A study undertaken by Gofton (1990) sheds some light on the phenomenon. Dorn (1983) has documented the governmental ambivalence towards drink. The market for alcohol is immensely profitable, and there has been a huge expansion in city centre drink retailing and leisure provision specifically targeted at younger consumers with high disposable incomes. Market forces are freely allowed to exploit this market, aided by central government's relaxation of licensing laws. But drink has always been seen as the vice of the working class, unable to control their appetites and regulate their lives. Social order is maintained by the dominant class policing and controlling the activity. Gofton took the view that drinkers do, in fact, police themselves, and that the *internal* set of rules and constraints that operate within a drinking group is far more important in determining behaviour than any externally applied restraint. Gofton's empirical data is supplied by young drinkers in the north-east of England and a contrast is made between old-style drinkers and the young. Although traditional drinking in the area involved heavy consumption, it was also invested with meaning. Drinkers in pubs were almost exclusively male, pubs were local and customers were loyal, drinking was social and value was placed on 'holding your drink'. Young drinkers cause concern to the older generation in the area more because of the way they drink rather than the fact that they drink too much. Leisure drinking for the young involves women too, at least until they marry and have children. Indeed women are central to the rituals that have evolved, rather than simply being tolerated within it. Pub forms have changed dramatically, neighbourhood loyalties have disintegrated, the young are mobile. A typical drinking bout takes place at weekends only and starts with a group between three and twenty gathering from the outskirts of the city where they live. They then move systematically around a circuit of pubs and clubs gaining members like a rolling snowball. Each visit may only last about twenty minutes. Each place is overcrowded and noisy. The atmosphere and style of each venue is very important to its customers. This is reflected both in the designer drinks consumed by young men and young women and by the fact that the whole circuit is dominated by courtship. Both men and women are on the lookout for 'talent' in the spots they visit.

These trappings are all-important, but what distances young drinkers too from their older counterparts is their attitudes to drunkenness. Younger drinkers seem less concerned with staying in control; many deliberately drink to get drunk:

> Many see alcohol as a major mood-altering drug, and both seek to expect to get drunk in the course of a weekend session ... The range of drink consumed, and their manner of consumption indicates clearly that young drinkers see it this way. Many said they drank 'for strong effect', and that they would choose a drink because of its potency. (Gofton, 1990, p.37)

Gofton looks at the function of drinking in the leisure lives of these two age groups. For the traditional drinkers, leisure time drinking is almost a celebration of the old working-class values of community, masculinity, social order. For the young drinkers leisure is seen as transformative and magical rather than reinforcing an existing lifestyle. Drink, for the young is a means of making a shift into a world of heightened sensations.

The present moral panic over lager louts is essentially about control and lawlessness, 'the latest version of a perennial problem' (Gofton, 1990, p.38), rather than about health. What is clear is that health education aimed at young people on the subject of alcohol consumption has to attack the very fundamental changes identified both in patterns of drinking and reasons for drunkenness.

Recreational drug use: into the Pleasuredome

An article by Fraser *et al.* (1991) based on work with a small section of Brighton's population, highlights another aspect of youth culture, namely attitudes to recreational drug use.

Ecstasy is a 'recreational' drug. It is seen mainly as a part of what has been known as the acid-house party scene which came about in the early 1980s. The culture has now spread throughout Britain. Newcombe, in a 1991 study, estimated that, at that time, in north-west England around 20,000 young people attended raves each weekend. It is argued that the rave scene is, potentially, a high-risk situation for users of 'E' in that many of them are young and new to the world of drug-taking and, consequently, have only limited knowledge of the drug or of how to cope with it on the basis of experience. Newcombe indicates that those who dominated the 'rave' scene are, in the main, working-class young adults. What differentiates this scene, however, from other youth cultures is the fact that group membership and shared beliefs don't figure very highly. Another interesting finding and different to many other youth scenes, is that there is an integration of young people of different ages, social backgrounds, race and sub-cultures. While much of the increase in attendance at 'rave' clubs is of young teenagers, Rietveld (1991) has noted that many of the key figures in this scene are people in their late twenties and early thirties. What Rietveld had identified in terms of the development of the 'rave' scene is that:

> Rather than fading away, between 1988 and 1989 the rave scene changed its status from cliquey, mutating underground sub-culture to a more socially diverse stable and consumerist popular leisure culture, blurring the boundaries between such previously disparate groups as football fans and various pop music 'tribes'. (Rietveld, 1991, p.3)

55

The attractions of 'raves' for young people amount to a heady cocktail of special music, buying new clothes, the thrill of secret locations and outwitting the police, an esoteric vocabulary to exclude the uninitiated, and a 'safe', 'party' drug which enables them to dance through the night and which allegedly heightens sexual excitement and performance. Unfortunately the number of deaths at 'raves' – fortunately very few – points towards risks related to excessive stresses on the cardio-vascular system associated with dehydration, liver damage and the use of impure 'fake' drugs cut with other substances.

The 'Pleasuredome' was the researchers' nickname for the entertainment centre of Brighton. As in Gofton's (1990) study, we are looking at a city or town centre location turned over at night to leisure consumption, and targeted specifically at young people, with boutiques, style pubs, wine bars, live music venues, fast food outlets and amusement arcades. Use of drugs was considered by the young people who frequented this area to be as valid a component of their leisure as drink, choice of friends or music and dress style. Workers at a drug advisory and information service working nearby (DAIS) shed some light on the phenomenon as they picked up the casualties. Most young people who referred themselves to the service were suffering from the side-effects of stimulant or hallucinogenic drugs, rather than being the traditional 'junkie'. One DAIS worker described them as 'a different and nicer type of drug user'. An examination of the DAIS records showed that most of the casualties fell within a very narrow age bracket (18 to 22). Men's use of the drugs clearly proved more problematic, even though equal numbers of women frequented the area. Almost all of the casualties were in employment or in further education and lived at home with parents. The concomitant of this was that though their actual incomes were not necessarily very high, their living expenses were small and they had relatively large disposable incomes for leisure.

Most thus lived quiet 'normal' lives at home for the rest of the week, bingeing at weekends only in association with peer group leisure activities. They were 'dedicated polyabusers', using not one drug but a whole range of different drugs concurrently. Cannabis, ecstasy, amphetamine sulphate, and LSD, all washed down with excessive levels of alcohol, form a potent cocktail. The reasons for taking such a mixture are, as in the case of Gofton's drinkers, to get high as quickly as possible in order to separate a magic world of leisure from the humdrum lives of mid-week. Characteristically, they saw themselves and their drug use as unproblematic, believing that the problem drug-takers were heroin users. However, a quarter of those reporting to DAIS had injected amphetamine and of these nearly half admitted sharing syringes. Such drug use is also clearly associated with unsafe and unprotected sex. Fraser *et al.* point to the fact that such a group of young people clearly see traditional anti-drugs campaigns as irrelevant. The interventions planned in the local area take account of the leisure context of such drug use by advertising the information and counselling service in local entertainment magazines, listings and even on club coasters. The chief message of the intervention revolves around harm reduction. Users are advised to take one drug at a time, monitor their own symptoms and to avoid sexual intercourse when stoned. The peer group is obviously an extremely important factor in this whole equation, encouraging individuals into 'a kind of stylised recklessness' (Fraser *et al.*, 1991, p.13). Infiltration of the peer group may thus be a key in any health intervention strategy and attempts need to be made to educate 15- and 16-year-olds, the 'apprentice' group, now standing in the wings and waiting to enter the scene. Klee (1991) reinforces this message in comparing young amphetamine users with heroin users:

> For example, the extent of sharing needles and syringes was greater. Motivations were different too. Sharing was not a consequence of desperation for an injection when experiencing withdrawal symptoms. The sharing of amphetamine users tended to relate to group involvement and the norms associated with it, in a much more pronounced way than was the case with heroin users. They were not only a more sociable group, they were also considerably more sexually active.   (Klee, 1991, p.3)

Coffield (1992) summarizes the difficulties which face health educators in relation to drug use. Epidemiological figures may show low levels of use of 'hard' substances, like heroin and cocaine, but the infiltration of drug use into some young people's leisure lifestyles is evident:

> Drug-taking, for those involved, is not an isolated aspect of young people's lives but is one of a number of activities like listening to music, drinking beer and talking to the opposite sex which are part and parcel of growing up for an increasing number of young adults. Drug use and pop culture are inextricably connected in the minds of all these young people and that is exactly its attraction. They see it as a world apart which they, and they alone, understand and into which they can pour their hopes, fears and creativity without worrying about interference from uncomprehending adults.   (Coffield, 1992, p.35)

Solvent use on a council estate

This account of a gang of 'sniffers' comes from a study carried out in north London in the mid-1980s (O'Bryan, 1989). Those who work on these problems with young people will recognize the account as fairly typical of what is happening in many city areas. Again, it identifies health concerns within lifestyle issues and makes the point that health education interventions have to tackle the issue – in this case, solvent abuse – according to the meaning and role it has for participants. At the time of the study local residents, youth workers and so on had become alarmed at the 'wave' of glue-sniffing that had washed in on the estate, though it was known that neighbouring estates had been affected earlier. All the solvent users were boys of around 14. Little sniffing was done in female company; in fact, these seemed to be boys who were particularly awkward with girls. Girls anyway are not part of the culture of hanging about on the streets in which sniffing flourishes.

The 'gang' was only loosely constituted, though they identi-fied themselves by their smart 'casual' sportswear and by particular types of music (rap and beatbox). There were clear leaders among the group. When the 'wave' hit the estate large numbers of boys experimented with sniffing. Debate exists over the usual proportion of regular to experimental users. The ratio of one to five proposed by Cohen (1973) is probably closest to the truth. Cohen had suggested that experimenters tried sniffing anything from one to ten times before deciding to abstain. O'Bryan noticed, instead, a seasonal element defining the degree of use. Summer holidays, for instance, provided the perfect opportunity for experimentation, with time on the hands of the young people concerned and no weather restrictions on outdoor activities. Almost all experimental sniffing took place in groups. For the majority the school holidays signalled the end of the practice. For a core group, however, even the cold weather did not deter them and use moved from the group to individual settings. The core users soon switched from glue to butane gas canisters, partly because it was less easy for parents and teachers to detect and partly because local shopkeepers had acted to limit glue sales. Sniffing was also clearly associated both with petty theft, shoplifting and vandalism. This was only partly a functional association. That is, although they often shoplifted for butane gas, for instance, to keep themselves supplied, most of the thefts had nothing to do with the habit. Often the goods stolen would simply be picked over and thrown away as useless. The point of 'lifting' them in the first place had been for the 'buzz' or thrill to be had from taking chances. The core users were central in organizing and carrying out such acts. Reports from elsewhere confirm similar links between solvent use and delinquency (Biggs *et al.*, 1983; Masterson, 1979).

O'Bryan, reflecting on her observations of the solvent users picks out two themes, which will be of relevance in our discussions in ensuing chapters. The first is the importance of peer group pressure. Opinion leaders are the first to introduce substances. They define substance use as a test of courage, a badge of membership, and thus exert pressure on others to take part. A second theme drawn out by O'Bryan is the users' emphasis on a 'hard man' image. The masculinization of the activity echoes that of drinking and also of the problematic recreational drug users. Some health education interventions may actually serve to reinforce rather than diminish the attractiveness of such activities by depicting them as extremely risky or 'beyond the pale'. To implicate peer pressure or the cultivation of a 'macho' image as responsible for decisions to be part of this misusing group is not to deny, however, that substance misusers also derived considerable pleasure from using glue or gas. Ignoring this fact is like denying that smokers clearly gain a physical lift from their pattern of use, and such denial does nothing to help frame ways of approaching young people in a way that addresses the problem from where they stand.

Concluding remarks

These illuminative ethnographic studies provide insights into adolescent health issues from the young person's perspective – in contrast to the more adultist orientation of large-scale survey research – and should be seen as complementary to the questionnaire-based findings reported in the first half of this chapter. They also offer more 'coloured' snapshots of adolescents' lifestyles and health issues which illustrate in more specific detail the broader, more general backcloth picture of survey findings. Hence, the purposes of this chapter have been to highlight some of the findings on young people's health, and on the social contexts within which young people have to make decisions and choices on health issues. In doing so we have examined both quantitative and qualitative ethnographic studies together with a brief consideration of their strengths and limitations, and examined health within the framework of adolescent lifestyle development.

3 School health education: paradigms and perspectives

Introduction

In the previous two chapters we have looked at young people's development and transitions towards adult society, and at existing patterns in their health and risk-taking behaviours together with some consideration of the psycho-social implications of these behaviours. In this chapter and the next we move on to examine a number of issues and underlying theories and themes in relation to the education of young people on health matters in the school setting. Neither of these chapters aims to be comprehensive in their coverage or review of activity in these areas. Rather it is hoped that these sections will highlight some of the dilemmas currently abroad in the field of school health education by bringing together aspects of the academic research literature and practitioners' attempts to provide health education on the ground.

Working from what we know about the characteristics of adolescent development in cognitive, physical, affective and social dimensions (outlined in the earlier chapters) should we be able to prescribe an ideal curriculum which matches appropriate information, learning/teaching style and so on to the appropriate stage of development of the child? Many curricular developments in this area are based around such a model of proceeding. One might anticipate already that such an undertaking is likely to be fraught with problems and possibly doomed to failure. The number of variables to be built into the programme is too many, the scale of things we *don't* know about young people is still too vast, the individual differences between youngsters may be so great as to make any such ideal curriculum for aggregated groups a fantastic proposition. Despite this, many health education programmes are planned from just such a viewpoint – they are designed from the top down and reflect what we think young people should know and understand, given our adult judgement of their level of understanding and the types of problems or contexts they will encounter at different developmental stages.

Knowing something of the nature and development of children and knowing something about the principles of good health, it is still an uncomfortable job trying to bring the two together in some sort of educational programme on health issues. In the first part of this chapter the failure of health education to affect the behaviour or beliefs of many people (of all ages) is explained through a variety of theoretical models which are rehearsed briefly here.

If this top-down design approach often yields inadequate programmes, is there an alternative? Is it feasible to imagine, for instance, asking young people themselves to identify their needs? We examine the arguments for talking to young people about their own health education needs, and assess the problems and potential in this sort of activity. This leads us on to a discussion of what some have evoked as models of health education, but which might be more correctly characterized as competing paradigms of health education. The chapter then moves on to look at some of the curricular offerings currently in place. From what have these developed and on what principles are they based? How do they equate with the frameworks elucidated in the earlier sections of this chapter? The development of health education curricula over the last half century is of more than historical interest. The choice of topics that we teach, the 'menu' that we select on behalf of children, and the teaching styles that are evoked are all highly reflective of the paradigm in which we operate in respect of young people.

In many ways even the rhetoric of health education is full of paradox. There is dissonance between curricular aims and teaching method, for example. There is tension between the aims of health educators and the developing para-profession of health promotion. Can these differences be resolved so that the classroom can become an effective forum for the successful education of young people on health issues?

Putting learning into practice: a perennial problem

Measuring the effectiveness of school health education programmes is notoriously difficult. A rather limited definition of 'effectiveness' might be one that simply measures achievement against a pre-specified list of objectives. The danger in accepting this as an appropriate definition in these circumstances, however, is that it is all too easy to 'let the tail wag the dog', and thus to establish programmes which have objectives which are easy to meet or easy to measure. We might be justifiably suspicious about health education programmes which concentrate, for instance, only on improving knowledge levels – do young people know more at the end of this campaign than at the beginning about HIV or heart disease or the dangers of smoking? Our suspicions are justifiable because we have too much evidence from young people's own accounts (Hendry *et al.*, 1993b) and from scrutiny of the figures that improving knowledge alone will not lead to a change in behaviour.

Young people are no different to the rest of us in this respect, and there is a veritable industry in the development of theoretical models (Green, 1984) purporting to explain our reluctance to put into practice what we know to be right or good for us. A brief survey of these is included here.

From a health education perspective, many models which look at change in behaviour – including health-related behaviour – are not cyclical, but linear, and appear at first sight to be simple and straightforward, since they do not include any discussion about the presence or absence of any desire for change. The simplest form of model is one that could be characterized as a *knowledge–attitude–behaviour model* which states that if one simply provides *knowledge* about a health topic (for example, about the unhealthy effects of smoking), this will induce a negative *attitude* towards smoking, and a consequent change in *behaviour* (i.e. the teenager gives up smoking). Ignorance is thus seen as the basic deficit. Gray and Blythe (1979) are cynical about this type of simplistic thinking which, coupled with a lack of planning or evaluation, leads to the vast majority of health education projects failing. We need to look further, then, so as to attempt to understand how the process of choosing to make changes in adolescent health behaviour may actually work.

The 'why' of making changes in health behaviour suggests that consideration should be given to the belief and value systems of both the individual and the society in which he or she lives. The *health belief model* has been attributed to Becker (1984), and Tones *et al.* (1990) have summarized the key points of this model by suggesting that making a decision about a specific health-related behaviour has more chance of being successfully carried out if the following belief elements are present:

1. That the person believes him/herself to be susceptible to the disease or illness;
2. That the person believes the disease or illness is serious;
3. That the person believes the proposed healthy choice will be successful;
4. That the person believes that the benefits will outweigh the 'costs'.

In addition, the health belief model suggests that a generally positive attitude to health (as shown by the individual often making healthy choices in other areas of life), and the presence of a trigger as a 'cue to action' are also necessary for the healthy choice to be made. The health belief model is somewhat limited in that it looks at disease prevention rather than taking an overall positive health promotion perspective. While it rightly brings into reckoning the seriousness of and susceptibility to illness like cancer and coronary heart disease, the health belief model concentrates on the absence of disease, rather than operating from a perspective of general well-being.

Morgan *et al.* (1985) have pointed out that the health belief model only explains a small amount of compliant health behaviour. They discuss health and illness behaviour from a collectivist as well as individual viewpoint. Belonging to a certain social or ethnic group, with its own 'norms' and values, they argue, will have an effect upon the health of individuals in that community. These social factors have a powerful effect in terms of influencing an individual's professional help-seeking behaviour, and are likely to be significantly different in a teenage sub-culture. Fishbein and Ajzen (1985) develop these thoughts as the *theory of reasoned action*. In separating beliefs from attitudes, they suggest that the degree of influence of 'significant others' – or chance events – in the individual's life is likely to be critical in predicting whether or not the decision will be acted upon.

The *health action model* is described by its originator as a 'mapping model', which is capable of absorbing both the health belief model and Fishbein's theory of reasoned action (Tones *et al.*, 1990). The model examines the interaction of: (a) *cognitive factors* (knowledge, skills and beliefs, including beliefs about how we feel about ourselves), (b) *motivating factors* (values, attitudes and drives), and (c) the *influence of the social norms* of the community we live in, which all are associated with behavioural intention. All these factors influence the balance between the conscious desire for change and the unconscious desire to avoid change, and suggest, to a lesser or greater extent, whether or not the behavioural change is actually contemplated.

The health action model begins by asking the same questions concerning beliefs as the health belief model, but then goes on to ask also about beliefs that one holds about oneself. A high sense of self-esteem and self-worth is seen as a very positive factor in making a healthy choice, since these attributes are directly associated with assertiveness and self-empowerment (Temple and Robson, 1991) – a belief in one's own ability to carry out a specific healthy action (Tones *et al.*, 1990). While knowledge alone is not enough, as we have seen in the knowledge–attitude–behaviour model, it is still a key

65

cognitive component in the health action model, and our mapping of likely health behaviour.

Baron and Brown (1991), in America, have argued that schools have neglected the metacognitive skill of decision-making, an area that some educators might call critical thinking. They propose a number of specific programmes for making decision-making an important educational focus. For example, they outline a GOFER curriculum, (i.e. Goals, Options, Facts, Effects and Review). Another decision-making process is the GOOP (Goals, Options, Outcomes and Probabilities). These programmes attempt to provide pupils with training in critical thinking that allows them to simplify complex problems. Young people need to be encouraged to understand cause, effect and consequences and to be helped to understand the strategies that lead to effective decision-making not only in the cognitive sphere but in social contexts too. We know from the work of Inhelder and Piaget (1958) and Kohlberg (1969) that young people strive in many sectors of their lives towards the level of intellectual reasoning that enables them to objectify and make reasonably rational decisions. Various studies have shown that young people's abilities to reason logically, to take responsibility for their actions and to make decisions is sometimes flawed and requires adult counselling and mentoring.

The motivation system describes a complex of attitudes and values which interact to determine whether or not the individual will be favourably disposed towards making the change. Values are acquired through socialization, so it may well be that an adolescent may value the company of her or his friends, who happen to be smokers, more than her or his desire to make a healthy choice to live in a smoke-free environment and so improve her or his health. She or he may also be inclined towards a fatalistic view of health ('if it happens, it happens'), though, as Pill and Stott (1985) have pointed out, fatalism and a positive attitude towards making lifestyle changes are not necessarily contradictory positions. The competent adolescent then should possess, firstly, an awareness and ability to reflect in a wide variety of life situations, and secondly, an under-standing of personal orientation to social contexts and settings that give the skills to take responsibility in 'action and decision-making'.

Cultural, sub-cultural and group pressures play as much of a role as individual psychology in deciding whether or not a healthy choice is made as Fishbein and Ajzen's theory makes clear. They obviously influence the values an individual may hold. Certain decisions about health (for example, deciding to seek psychiatric help or to live openly as a homosexual) may well be contentious in the eyes of many of one's peers. Peer pressure is important at any age, but particularly so in adolescence. Stigma, however, does to some extent imply a passive agreement to be stigmatized for acting in a certain 'abnormal' way. An autonomous person, who is someone capable of awareness, spontaneity and intimacy, with a high level of self-esteem, is likely to resist pressures to stigmatize her or him for behaving in the way she or he has decided upon. In this case, the effect of normative pressures would be minimal. This person may be said to have both a strong self-image and self-concept (Schools Council Health Education Project, 1982), and also a positive internal locus of control (Head, 1987; Eachus, 1991; Peterson and Stunkard, 1989). Hence, we can conclude that it is she or he – rather than significant others or chance events – who is in charge of making choices and changes in her or his life, though this is not to deny the role of significant powerful others in our lives.

Problematizing youth health: politics and moral panics

Thus far we have described a set of explanatory models which aim to explain some of the dissonance between our knowledge and our actions on health. Such models also serve to provide key pointers for health educationalists about which are the optimal conditions which assist people in making reasonable choices about their own health. These models, however, are not specific to youth. They explain why adults eat the wrong

food, take a drink too many or fail to exercise as well as
(or perhaps better than) they explain why young people
are attracted to drug use or fail to use condoms when having
sex.

One of the characteristics of health education aimed at
young people, however, is the extent to which the added ingredi-
ent of 'youth' seems to change the general agenda. We have
looked in the first section of this book, for instance, at young
people's propensity for risk-taking. Elkind (1984) has
described the perceived invulnerability of young people as the
Personal Fable and others have gone on to explore both the
positive and negative consequences of this Personal Fable
(Jack 1989; Irwin and Millstein 1986).

A further dimension of the argument of particular importance concerns the observation by Jessor (1987 and 1991) that
such risk-taking behaviours and the rationale for them is far
from homogeneous, but rather reflects the variety of socio-
economic and micro-cultural backgrounds of young people:

> Overall the empirical evidence supports the existence of organised
> patterns of adolescent risk behaviour. These structures of behav-
> iours, taken together, reflect an adolescent's way of being in the
> world ... Part of the answer probably lies in the social ecology of
> adolescent life, an ecology that provides socially-organised oppor-
> tunities to learn risk behaviours together and normative
> expectations that they be performed together.   (Jessor, 1991; p.9)

A lot of work needs to be done to expand the existing evidence
on this heterogeneity of experience from young people's own
perspective (Hendry *et al.*, 1991 and 1993b; Glendinning *et
al.*, 1992).

Considerable attention has been paid in recent years to the
fact that most agendas for health education (whether through
the formal curriculum or through agencies like the health
promotion departments and local health boards or national
organizations like the Health Education Authority and the
Health Education Board for Scotland) are set by adults.
Moreover they are set by adults who tend to problematize

youth. Rarely are young people themselves consulted about their priorities or needs.

Tilford (1992) notes 'that young people's own views of their health concerns do not entirely equate with those of adults' and she points to the work of Balding (1987) and Friedman (1989) in support of this statement. More emphasis has been given to this point in a World Health Organization (WHO) document (1989) on the health of youth. Levin (1989), in discussing this, states that it is essential, therefore, that policy formulation be fundamentally a public process with continuous inputs from young people as well as those who claim to represent them.

Such ideas have been advocated strongly in relation to the relatively new field of health education for young people on the topic of HIV/AIDS. Aggleton *et al.* (1992), for instance, comment that the concept of participation is central to much youth work, as well as those styles of health promotion which go beyond the simple provision of information. In their view, a participatory needs assessment should become a prerequisite for future work with young people. They feel that focus group work involving young people directly in the agenda-setting process and leading to the identification of intervention priorities, should precede any local HIV/AIDS health promotion initiative. Thus while they feel that the view of teachers, parents, youth leaders and other adults may be sought, they are convinced that these views should never be afforded priority over the express needs of young people themselves.

This point has been brought to a finer focus within Scotland recently by the publication of the draft Scottish Agenda for Children by the Children's Rights Development Unit (CRDU, 1994). Taking as one of its main themes 'Health and Health Care services', the Agenda attempts to translate the general recommendations of the United Nations Convention on the Rights of the Child (to which Britain is a signatory) into a Scottish policy context. In examining children's rights within the health context, the Agenda draws attention to Article 12 of the UN Convention which makes it clear that children and young people have the right to express their views, and to have those views taken into account.

These themes find echoes in both the research literature and in social legislation that emphasizes young people's rights and 'citizenship'. The Children Act of 1989 (HMSO, 1989) undoubtedly brought to the forefront discussions about young people's issues and their rights to have a voice in relation to their own welfare in many spheres. The work of Jones and Wallace (1992), at a theoretical level, has again emphasized young people's need to have better rights as citizens if they are to develop as responsible members of the community. They state:

> The imposition of dependency status on many young people who in other historical or social circumstances might be able to live independent lives, takes away adult responsibility and places young people under the legal control of their parents. Their rights to freedom and self-determination are thus restricted. So too are their responsibilities. Thus, at a time when both independence and responsibilities should be increasing, they are not. Yet rights and responsibilities are inextricably linked...
>
> (Jones and Wallace, 1992, p.154)

However, some of the rationale for this new interest in listening to young people's views must lie in the recognition that existing health education messages and interventions are increasingly shown to have little impact on the actual behaviour of large segments of the young population. Smoking rates among young people demonstrate a hard core of smokers resistant to every form of media campaign, for example, and more young women seem to be attracted to smoking than ever. Information campaigns about HIV are shown to raise knowledge levels, yet risky sexual behaviours are still commonplace. Drug culture seems to embed itself more firmly among young people whether health promoters 'say no' or seek a harm minimization approach.

At the root of it all, however, it is likely that too much of what we thrust at young people in the way of education and information about their health reflects our adult agendas, our concerns as parents, as experts, as professionals. What is missing is any honesty about why we have set the agenda in this way and whether it bears any similarity to young people's own concerns.

In relation to the first of these it is clear that many adult agendas for young people's health rest on a bedrock of concern over social control. Much of this reflects the moral panics that seem to overtake society at times of uncertainty. Does the current scapegoating of young people and of single parents and their putative association with poor child-rearing reflect a conscious or unconscious desire to find a set of victims on which to deflect society's anger or frustration with a much broader malaise which is about social decline and lack of direction?

> Societies appear subject, every now and then, to periods of moral panic. A condition, episode, person or group of persons emerges to become defined as a threat to societal values and interests; its nature is presented in a stylised and stereotypical fashion by the media. Sometimes the object of the panic is quite novel and at other times it is something which has been in existence long enough, but suddenly appears in the limelight. Sometimes the panic passes over and is forgotten, except in folklore and collective memory; at other times it has more serious and long-lasting repercussions and might produce such changes as those in legal and social policy or even in the way that society conceives itself. (Cohen, 1972, p.14)

Griffin's recent work (1993) highlights the extent to which work on adolescence has concentrated on 'troubled youth'. She notes how many teenage activities are problematized, how many analyses centre around blaming young people and then 'treating' them. Education is singled out for its tendency to view young people as 'deficient' in some way. They are either deficient in knowledge (which research has shown is often far from true), or they are deficient in rationality (whereas it is the assumption that we all act on a rational basis that is deficient). Griffin's work is a plea for us to deconstruct the theoretical frameworks and sets of assumptions through which we tend to view young people's health beliefs and to examine instead the explanations and rationale that young people themselves hold for their actions and beliefs.

Testing the water: what do young people think about their health?

If health education must be salient, then, and reflect young people's own concerns, how are we, either as researchers or teachers (or perhaps as teacher-researchers) to gather information on their needs and requirements?

One of the principal difficulties involved in assessing young people's health beliefs from a researcher's point of view rests in the methodological problems encountered. Farquhar (1990) has pointed to the lack of development of methods for exploration with young people on health topics (but see Backett and Alexander, 1989 and Williams *et al.*, 1989a and 1989b, for example), and has rehearsed some of the practical problems as well as the theoretical ones which jeopardize the validity of much such research.

It is now commonplace to reflect on how an imbalance of power in an interview setting, for instance, may compromise the validity of the account obtained. The problem exists in all research carried out by this method, for the interviewer/interviewee relationship almost always reflects an asymmetry of power, often exacerbated by a social class differential. With young people, however, this imbalance is particularly acute, since the interview relationship often mimics the usual social relationships between adults and children. Farquhar comments:

> Children will already have direct experience of unequal power relationships with a variety of adults. They will have learnt, through experience, both the explicit and implicit rules which govern adult-child relationships in schools, particularly teacher-child relationships, and will bring this knowledge and experience to bear on their relationships with unfamiliar adults who enter this context.
> (Farquhar, 1990, p.23)

A further dimension to this problem is discussed by Backett and Alexander (1989), who note that a particular problem involved in interviewing children comes in disentangling the 'public' and 'private' accounts that children are prepared to give. Many research techniques, for example, encourage children to reproduce messages that they have absorbed from teachers, from television or from other forms of media campaign. Reproduction of such 'public' messages, however, gives little insight into the 'private' logic and reasoning that guides children's beliefs, values and actions.

It is for these reasons that research has surprisingly little to tell us about how young people reason in relation to their health. We know too little about how they define health, how they negotiate health issues in relation to families (though see Brannen *et al.*, 1994) and to friends, and how their cognition on these topics changes as they advance through childhood and puberty. If researchers find it so difficult to access young people's views and perspectives, how then are teachers and curriculum planners supposed to build such insights into their own work?

Perhaps the answer lies at several levels. Many schools, for instance, now undertake a deliberate audit of health behaviours and beliefs among their pupils. Sometimes this is the work of a single person or group acting on their own initiative within a school. Often the need for such an exercise may only become clear when a particular panic hits the community over under-age drinking or solvent use, for instance. Few settings could be worse for a piece of exploratory research. One particular issue is brought to the forefront at the expense of a broader view of health, pupils and parents are so keyed up about the issue that sensitivities are heightened and true responses may be hard to obtain. Local media may hound the school, scenting a scandal.

Some schools or authorities have, however, decided to approach the problem in a more rational and measured way. Thus a health audit might be carried out as part of a whole-school review of policy and practice on health education, and problem issues would then be embedded in a much more holistic view of young people's health concerns. Some education authorities have entered into partnerships with local health boards to carry out such exploratory work. Thus, for instance, a number of local health boards in Scotland (either through the Health Promotion Department or the Department of Public Health Medicine) have undertaken health and lifestyle surveys of young people in their local schools. Great care has been taken in these exercises to preserve confidentiality and to take cognizance of schools' need to handle such data carefully. Thus, for example, a survey undertaken by Forth Valley Health Board using a standard questionnaire which is commercially available produced a summary report of aggregated data for the whole health board area (Forth Valley Health Board, 1994) but data for each school was not published and was only available for inspection by each school's senior management team, which then had the choice of how to use the information. Schools could compare their results with the aggregated summary for the whole region, or with national data made available by the unit which analysed the data on the Health Board's behalf. Some schools were brave enough to band together to compare results for adjacent geographical areas.

Such exercises can reveal a lot in terms of pupils' levels of knowledge and activity and may help to suggest areas where health education could be targeted more specifically, but they suffer from the drawback noted before that children are asked to respond in relation to an agenda defined by adults. The questions to which they supply responses may not represent the issues of concern to them.

An alternative approach might be to encourage young people themselves to carry out an audit of health knowledge within their own environment as part of their course work in health eduation. Handled carefully the product might be a questionnaire which identified more apposite topics in language which was more user-friendly. There would be no comparative base, of course, in a study undertaken in this way, unless schools pooled the needs they identified.

An alternative form is simply to adopt a style of teaching which gears itself to listening as much as it does to instructing. It is not uncommon to find health education programmes which advocate small group work, which emphasize the need for young people to find a true voice in these where their confidences are respected, and in which the concerns of the young people themselves can be built into a flexible programme. Such operating principles run so counter to most of the other operations of the curriculum, however, that they sometimes require fundamental gearing of the system if they are to happen. These problems are referred to again in a later section. Many teachers find their way around them, as a Tayside document shows (Tayside Regional Council, 1993), by simple devices or exercises such as prioritizing 'card sorts', 'draw and write', sentence completion, group discussion, contributions placed anonymously in a suggestion box and so on. The principle is a simple one: we should never assume that we know already what young people know, or that we know what they want and need to know.

Consideration of this issue highlights the very different paradigms within which health education can operate within schools, and we go on to examine this in the next section.

Informed or empowered: how should young people be involved?

Given the theoretical models which indicate the best conditions under which knowledge might be transferred into behaviour, and given some understanding of young people's own priorities and saliences with regard to their health, how then should we organize teaching and learning in school health education?

Again the literature presents us with a set of what are often called 'models' of health education, though they bear the characteristics of competing paradigms (Kuhn, 1962), in that they determine both the criteria according to which one selects and defines problems and the methods by which one researches or teaches about them.

We look briefly now at the theoretical formulation of these models before going on to describe how they have been expressed in the actual curriculum of our schools.

The *information-giving model* of health education has been the traditionally dominant form developed in health education, fitting most easily into bio-medical definitions of health and illness. It is further characterized by Tones *et al.* (1990) as a 'preventive' type mode. It is a model comfortably used in many formal educational settings, focusing as it does on the need for the individual to change rather than the society or institution. The role of the educator is seen to be the passing on of information to a rational audience who will then internalize the messages and act accordingly. Thus information is assumed to be objective and unproblematic. It is assumed that those rejecting or missing the 'messages' are 'deficient' in some way.

Gatherer (1979) concluded that messages based on this method are unsuccessful and even counter-productive at a mass level, though they may be more successful at a micro-level within groups who feel motivated to change their behaviour. This has been amplified in relation to work on tobacco education (Gillies, 1989), alcohol education (Plant and Stuart, 1984; Bagnall, 1989) and powerfully highlighted in relation to health education carried out in the climate of AIDS (Aggleton, 1989; Clift *et al.*, 1989; Ingham *et al.*, 1992). The HIV/AIDS crisis has highlighted the way that information that is not linked to a wider set of strategies may have distorting consequences: Aggleton (1989), for example, found that while levels of knowledge about dangers may be increased, anxiety and confusion may interfere with messages about safer practices. Since such messages are, by their nature, simplified, groups and individuals who do not fit into the mainstream may be further alientated and marginalized. As Clift *et al.* (1989) have suggested, what constitutes safe sexual practice may be at odds with what constitutes safer educational content. Thus, taken-for-granted notions about the nature of sexuality and sexual behaviour have become issues for debate and have pointed up the ways in which this model, far from transmitting unproblematic messages, has tended to reinforce dominant ideological themes of sexual behaviour. The Women Risk Aids Project papers (Holland *et al.* 1990a and 1990b), based on research carried out in Manchester and London, have examined how this has been particularly clear in relation to the difficulties facing young women in negotiating sexual encounters, given the contradictory expectations about their role.

A number of surveys of the knowledge, beliefs and understanding of young people in relation to HIV/AIDS have clearly identified that the acquisition of knowledge is only one of a range of factors which will affect future behaviour (Hastings and Scott, 1988; Holland *et al.*, 1990a and 1990b; Aggleton and Homans, 1988; Wight, 1990).

Past experience of alcohol and drugs education programmes based on this model has similarly demonstrated that these can have counter-productive effects in stimulating interest rather than discouraging use (Bagnall, 1989). Bagnall argues the need for initiatives which take account of social contexts since these sorts of initiatives overwhelmingly and characteristically disregard the socio-political roots of ill-health. Tones *et al.* (1990) use the powerful analogy of the drowning man in the river. Health education of this type is concerned only with fishing people out of the water downstream. There is no interest in what is going on upstream to precipitate bodies into the water in this fashion.

The *self-empowerment* or *person-centred approach* has gained increasing currency in recent years and is in direct contrast to the previous model which views lay beliefs as unhelpful or even misleading. This approach recognizes that such beliefs and experiences have an important role in how people understand and make sense of the processes of health. Skills-based education aimed at providing people with resources to make positive decisions has been particularly popular in the construction of 'packs' aimed at schools. It assumes that through building up self-esteem and confidence, individuals will be in a better position to make positive decisions about their health and to develop the skills to act on these. Mechanisms like assertiveness training, self-help initiatives and group work where the educator acts as a resource for the group, are key approaches. The provision of information on which to base informed choice is important, but the educator is no longer the 'expert' and repository of knowledge, but is rather a facilitator who can help individuals recognize their potential. This model has overtones of therapy, focusing on the removal of 'blocks' and anxieties, having its origins in the treatment of particular problems such as phobias.

The emphasis on 'private' accounts and centralizing of lay beliefs about health represents a move to recognizing the importance of subjective understandings. However, it has severe limitations if it remains the only level of intervention or if the conditions which create the problem in the first place remain unchanged, as Aggleton (1989) points out. Tones *et al.*'s (1990) analogy of the drowning man springs to mind again. Perhaps with this model we are teaching him better swimming skills, but the essential problem further upstream remains unchallenged. By focusing on the individual, such an educational programme may set people up to fail, if particular standards cannot be met. For instance, it can lapse into a 'blame the victim' approach if it merely reinforces the belief that the individual has responsibility for her own health without reference to the overall context. For example, young women may recognize the importance of using contraception, may even be able to negotiate this with a partner, but may be unable to follow it through in relation to getting access to condoms at a local clinic.

Alternatives to these models can be found in the form of *community development approaches*, discussed more fully in Chapter 5, and often cited as falling under the umbrella of 'health promotion'. Broadly, health promotion locates health education as one process within a holistic definition of health.

It explicitly recognizes that social, political and economic factors are factors in health and in so doing, highlights the limitations of traditional health education. It is inextricably bound up with community development approaches. The WHO describes it as the growth of health promotion built on public rather than medical-professional interest, and linked to a growing interest among the general public in positive health, in personal growth and in community development.

However, the breadth of the term and experience of the reality has led to criticisms that it is simply concerned with presenting a glossy image and 'number crunching' campaigns which have little to do with genuine community development. A number of health promotion initiatives have been organized as an attempt to deal with those who have traditionally resisted health education messages. Often these have been in relation to specific campaigns to raise awareness about issues identified as important by professionals. For example, 'fun' ways have been devised of encouraging the public to join in a range of activities. Large halls are hired where health educators and other professionals can set out their stalls and perhaps offer the chance to measure weight, heart rate etc. In this way it is hoped to recreate the 'spirit of community' by bringing people together in the belief that this will create a sense of belonging assumed to be lost in modern urban life. Such an approach has undoubted merit in redressing the image of health as boring and negative, but it is doubtful whether it reaches a population not already clued in to the health messages it puts across. Genuine consultation within community groups in this top-down model remains minimal and the content of the education accordingly remains at an information-giving level. Operating on such a large scale, the community appealed to may be a reality only in the health educator's mind with little evidence of a self-critical approach to the delivery of services or organization of the work.

Community development models, on the other hand, aim to involve people in the design and structure of their education based on a need or issue identified by a group often meeting in a neighbourhood or around an interest. This may include elements of the self-empowerment model but will also focus on collective solutions. Such groups often adopt a critical approach to existing provision and may themselves devise ways of providing a service or of lobbying the relevant authorities to meet the need. Some groups will also adopt a confrontational role with professional groups and policy-makers. Others concentrate on offering alternative models of existing provision which respond more sensitively and effectively to consumers. Tones *et al.* (1990) characterize this form of health education as a *radical-political model*. To refer again to the drowning man analogy, the emphasis has now shifted upstream within this model, as an attempt is made to get at the roots of ill-health.

The impact of the women's movement in particular has been powerful at community level in bringing issues hitherto seen as 'private' into public debate. A further example comes from another area of health education. In their analysis of school smoking education programmes, for instance, Nutbeam *et al.* (1993) compared the failure of the Family Smoking Education Project in the UK with its success in Norway. While there were methodological differences which made an exact comparison difficult, Nutbeam contrasts the Norwegian survey where there was a backdrop of 'a consistent decrease in the prevalence of smoking amongst young people in the country and comprehensive controls on the price, availability and promotion of tobacco products', with the UK, where 'cigarettes are still relatively easy to obtain ... legislation to restrict sales is largely ineffective ... and young people's purchasing patterns can be influenced by advertising and tobacco advertising of sports' (p.106). Since one of the *Health of the Nation* (DoH, 1992) targets specifically concerns smoking and young people, any Health Action Model analysis of action towards meeting this target is likely to suggest that teachers and other health educators need to spend time advocating changes in policy, such as pressing for a ban on cigarette advertising, alongside their implementing smoking education programmes.

So you have to change society before you can change people? I'm perfectly sure about that. That doesn't obliterate the concept of personal responsibility, but you can only have responsibility if the environment permits or encourages it. (Soper, 1993, p.3)

The development of community-based health groups falls into this category, organizing as they do around an issue and providing a forum for exchange of experience, ideas, information and support as well as developing a critical perspective on existing deficiencies in services. Planning groups may include women from both professional and community backgrounds who attempt to work on equal terms. The organization of 'well woman' days by some of these groups has resulted in a cross-section of women becoming involved in workshops and participating in the development of the groups.

The role of the educator within this process is complex, problematic and fraught with contradictions. The educator needs a range of skills in working with groups, a clear analysis of the aims and limitations of the piece of work and access to resources. The worker must tread a delicate path between encouraging participation by individuals in groups and refraining from creating dependency.

We turn now to an analysis of the ways in which these understandings about the links between knowledge, learning and action have been built into school curricula on health education.

A curricular problem

Health education occupies a paradoxical position within the curriculum. Students of the politics of curriculum will note with interest the high priority placed on the role of the school by government in raising the health standards and controlling the health behaviours of the nation's children. At the same time the pressures on the curriculum to expand attention to basic disciplines and to encompass a broad range of applied and technological subjects squeeze health education into a marginal slot.

Schools seem attractive places to people in government when planning campaigns to influence health behaviour. Within their walls schools gather (admittedly by compulsion) all the nation's children. Young people are a captive audience, held within structures designed to inculcate information and skills. Children, are, as we are often reminded, the future of the nation. Even if their parents are recalcitrant in their lust for nicotine or cholesterol-laden food, perhaps the chance exists with these children of catching their young impressionable minds before habits and attitudes are entrenched:

> In this area the most intimately personal and the widest social concerns intersect ... and the issues thrown up by these points of intersection are best dealt with, in our society, in the absence of any other appropriate public institution, in the personal and social education provided during the period of compulsory education.
>
> (White, 1991, p.399)

Teachers, of course, tend to view it all rather differently. They know only too well that children can go absent without leave even while physically on the premises. Lack of engagement with what is being taught allows many young people to process large chunks of information placed before them with as little involvement as postal workers sorting mail on a conveyor belt. It takes skilled and committed teaching to present material to young people in a way which is attractive and which will have impact. Teachers too are well aware that children are not empty jugs to be filled or clean sheets on which to be written. Their response to information or ideas is heavily driven by home background, and by the prejudices and preferences both of their immediate family and by the norms of their chosen peer group. Education which pays no attention to these existing structures and beliefs is almost not worth delivering.

Here then lie the roots of our paradox. The political drive to improve the nation's health is expressed in terms of goals and indices that will measure improvement outcomes. Schools seem economical and obvious structures through which to implement much of the education through which these improvements will be achieved. Once given the task, however, educators begin the spoiling function of bringing it down to reality. They point out that conveying knowledge alone is insufficient, that existing prejudices have to be challenged, that skills need to be developed, that programmes have to be rooted in young people's experience and be real and relevant to them. They have the authority of a range of research and theoretical developments outlined in the earlier sections of this chapter to support this stance. Health education thus becomes a political issue, laden with judgements and values, confronting and questioning practices and structures.

Tilford (1992), following Whitehead (1989), lists some of the contradictions that thus beset school health education:

(1) policies encouraging broadly based health education incorporating positive conceptions of mental, physical, and social health *BUT* direct government pressure from 1985 for 'crisis' education in schools on separate health problems;

(2) DES and other policies encouraging development of health education and personal and social education as essential parts of the curriculum *BUT* no place for these as core or foundation subjects in the National Curriculum;

(3) a broadening of the concept of sex education and its incorporation into wider health and personal education programmes *BUT* school governors given responsibility to decide if it should be included, and if so what and how;

(4) HMI encouragement of greater exploration of sensitive issues of homosexuality, contraception, and abortion *BUT* teachers advised not to give contraceptive advice to girls under 16 and restrictions imposed on discussions of homosexuality;

(5) schools increase health education in the formal curriculum *BUT* generally fail to develop and implement health-promotion policies for the school as a whole. Messages conveyed by the school environment and the school ethos contradict messages from the formal curriculum.   (Tilford, 1992, p.127)

The school's role as an agent in the improvement of the nation's health has a long pedigree, as Farley (1991) points out. The poor physical condition of recruits for the Boer War at the very end of the nineteenth century revealed the danger of the *laissez-faire* social policies of much of that period. The operation of market forces, that particular Victorian value now resurrected as a modern idiom, had left an industrial or working class which was often undernourished, and which suffered all the physical consequences of poor housing and ill-regulated working conditions. The growth of public health interventions in the form of the provision of better sanitation, programmes of inoculation and so on, did much to remove the depredations of infectious disease in the latter half of the nineteenth century. What remained were the diseases and illnesses that accompanied constitutions weakened by the impoverished conditions within which many people lived.

It is interesting to look at the concept of 'public health' as it developed then. Improving the nation's health was not then (as it is now) portrayed as an exercise to improve individual quality of life and enhance personal potential. Improving the health of the working classes was rather a necessary measure for the protection of other ranks in society (infectious disease often knew no social boundaries), and an economic necessity in terms of the development of the nation's resource (undernourished or tubercular soldiers or workers were hardly an asset). While many public health reformers were clearly motivated by Christian or strong humanitarian principles and valued the individual, the development of the health education movement may have been rooted in much more pragmatic principles.

One positive way of improving the condition of the poor was through education in better nutrition (through the introduction of domestic science as a school subject), and through the development of physical education, often pursued through complex drilling rituals which remind one of its origins as a remediation of military shortfalls.

There was, however, no overall co-ordination of health education within the curriculum for the first half of the twentieth century. Schools were left to follow and develop policies of their own. Characteristically the stress on subjects related to health and fitness was strongest in the types of schools and social areas where children were most seen to be at risk. Grammar schools showed little concern for their charges' health and devoted only minimal curricular time to it.

The advent of the 1960s, however, saw a rash of organized activity around curriculum development, and this encompassed health education too. The earliest of these initiatives (a collaborative project developed by the Schools Council for the Curriculum and Examinations and the Health Education Council) seems surprisingly modern in its assumptions and must have dropped like a bombshell into the tranquil waters of many school health education programmes at that time (Schools Council, 1977).

The Primary Schools Project, for children aged 5 to 13, concentrated on the development of an educational rationale for school health education. This was quite at odds with the mechanistic and pragmatic approach which previously characterized such work. It argued, for instance, that a main goal for such programmes should be the development of self-esteem and decision-making skills. The teaching of health topics was envisaged as an activity that would be taught through the medium of other curricular subjects such as art, language and so on, as much as a subject in its own right.

The rationale for the Secondary Schools Project was similar, though there was, for obvious reasons, less attention to the cross-curricular benefits of teaching. Farley (1991) notes that health education, perhaps unfettered by the disciplinary demands of more traditional subject areas, was often in the vanguard for the development of organizational change strategies and for promoting personal change in learners and teachers.

Health education undoubtedly gained status in the school curriculum at this period, and various articles in the practitioner press noted that it had 'moved into the mainstream' (Reid, 1981) or 'come of age' (Conley, 1978). To reinforce this notion that health education was innovatory and influential, Massey (1990) lists a stunning array of developments in the pastoral curriculum, in social education and so on which fed off and utilized the central concepts of health education, all of them focusing around the importance of fostering self-esteem and informed decision-making.

The advanced nature of this educational thinking was highlighted again in the 1980s when attention focused on the idea of health education being carried out within the context of a whole-school ethos which emphasized health – the health-promoting school concept. All aspects of the school environment, from the culinary offerings of the canteen to the smoking behaviour of teachers were to be audited and assessed in terms of their contribution to the message that young people received about health.

Farley (1991) notes that one of the outcomes (if not the progenitor) of these moves to the health-promoting school was the concurrent growth of health promotion as an arm of the health services dedicated to prevention rather than remediation. Within Scotland, for instance, this shift was marked by the establishment of the Scottish Health Education Group (SHEG) as part of the Common Services Agency to take forward work on health education in Scotland (SHHD, 1991). At the same time the Scottish Health Education Co-ordinating Committee was established. In the same year what became known as the SHAPE document (Scottish Health Authorities Priorities for the Eighties) was published (Scottish Health Service Planning Council, 1980). This emphasized the need for health service authorities to move more resources into prevention, and particularly into health promotion or education. While on one level one can see the partnership that arose from the developments as innovative in terms of intersectoral collaboration, it is also clear that they have in some senses detracted from the educational and veered towards the promotional, allowing schools to point to healthy tuckshops or mass physical jerks sessions in the school hall in aid of better heart health as the evidence of their commitment to health education.

Many of the efforts of health promotion are, however,

regressive in educational terms. They concentrate on the transmission of information (on the assumption that this will effect behaviour change). The message they deliver is homogeneous and takes no account of prior learning or knowledge or social circumstances. While one may welcome the alliance between educational and health service sectors on many grounds (not least for the additional resources that can be deployed within educational settings), there must be room for concern that these endeavours will emphasize the message rather than the medium, and that the attention to learning which characterized earlier curricular endeavours might be lost.

Even the introduction of health promotion rhetoric and of documents which emphasized the whole-school approach were wasted however where there was little managerial support for the development of this approach. The Scottish Consultative Committee on the Curriculum produced its booklet 'Promoting Good Health: Proposals for Action in Schools' in 1990. While reiterating the need for school health education to develop in young people skill in making choices and confirming the importance of a health-promoting ethos and environment, the report conceded that few Scottish schools provided the kind of programme which met their broad criteria (SCCC, 1990). The report called upon regional authorities to take the initiative by stating their policy on health education, but stressed that leadership should go beyond the statement of principle. Schools were exhorted to appoint a co-ordinator. Local authorities were urged to monitor such appointments and support developments. None of these recommendations was mandatory and studies show their implementation to have been very patchy (Hendry *et al.*, 1991). Devine *et al.* (1993), following a survey of Scottish schools, revealed that the existence of a local authority health education policy was particularly important for secondary schools. Where there was no regional policy, schools had made their own assumptions about the value and place of health education among competing claims and only 30 per cent of secondary schools had developed their own policy.

The year 1990 also saw the publication in England of guidance on health education from the National Curriculum Council. This followed growing concern about the possible fate of health education in schools once the provisions of the Education Reform Act came into being.

Donoghue (1991) notes that within these documents the wish is expressed that health education should not be seen as an additional subject in the curriculum. Many of the elements identified in the document should be taught through a variety of curricular areas and reinforced through the wider aspects of school life. Donoghue feels that in order for this not to be seen as a way of 'losing' health education, a variety of supporting documents are necessary to show teachers in other curricular areas how they might incorporate health education concerns, and training is also required in the use of teaching methods based on the active involvement of pupils.

Curricular development in Scotland has run largely in tandem with developments south of the border. The chief attainment outcome for the health education component is embedded in the National Guidelines for Environmental Studies and is seen to be 'healthy and safe living', attained through the study of three broad themes: looking after oneself; relationships; health and safety in the environment (SOED, 1993). 'Key features' describe activities to encourage pupils to develop a sense of responsibility for their own health and for the well-being of others at school, at home and in the wider environment. There are two 'strands' set, namely 'knowledge' and 'taking action on health', with attainment targets for each strand defined for levels A to E. In helping people to acquire knowledge, skills and understanding, it is essential that they are given the opportunity to participate actively in their own learning, through debate and discussion, through negotiation and investigation. The guidelines also encourage people to make connections between components of environmental studies and other areas of the 5 to 14 curriculum. For example, 'healthy and safe living' can be linked to aspects of expressive arts, religious and moral education and personal and social education.

In many respects these latest curricular documents on health education do not differ substantially from the earlier Schools Council work in the late 1970s in their emphasis on the cross-curricular nature of the issues, in their emphasis on building self-esteem and personal and interpersonal skills as a route to the achievement of long-term goals for better health, in their plan for a spiral syllabus in which issues are returned to at different stages with appropriately framed material and methods. Where they do differ they reflect changes in the education system more generally.

Among these changes of course is the imposition of a structured and graded curriculum with performance checks built into the system. It remains to be seen whether this results in an overemphasis on knowledge or information at the expense of the development of skills and qualities which are harder to evaluate.

It will also be interesting to observe over the next few years whether the advent of the 'new managerialism' in schools (Fairley and Patterson, 1995) will have an impact on the character of school health education. The health-promoting school movement, innocent in its origins as an attempt to instil a more holistic approach to health in the school context may yet be hijacked as part of the audit of school ethos, or used as a marketing ploy as schools move into a competitive mode within certain areas. The devolution of school budgets may also be the harbinger of change for school health education. Will the need to count costs and justify expenditure result in a greater readiness on the part of schools to enter into alliances with other agencies who will pay or contribute resource to their health education programme? Does this signal a vast opportunity for health promotion to move into formal education in a big way, and what will be the impact of this development on school curricula?

For now such issues are merely speculation. What we can say in summary, however, is that the official curriculum for health education expressed through the formal documents and through national guidelines is now very firmly in the mould of individual empowerment, as characterized earlier in this chapter. Such documents spurn the simplistic model of information-giving, but equally they eschew discussion of fundamental inequalities in health on the whole and certainly do not seek to empower people collectively to challenge or change the structural conditions which determine their well-being and health. Perhaps it is unrealistic to expect that they might? We continue this debate in the next chapter, as we start to unravel some of the professional responsibilities that teachers face as health educators and look at some of the problems that they face in this role.

4 Teaching and learning about health in schools

Introduction

We have in the previous chapter explored what the official position is with regard to national curricula for health education and examined briefly how these relate to theoretical models of learning in health, and also to prevailing paradigms about health education in general. What turns up in official curricula and policy statements and guidelines may be very different, however, from what is going on in the classroom. Do the learning and teaching interchanges in classrooms today reflect the prevailing paradigm or do they depart from it significantly?

In this chapter we look at some of the issues surrounding how health education is actually taught in classrooms. In doing this we rely heavily on our own studies carried out with teachers and with other educators in the field concerning the specific issue of health education relating to sexuality and drug misuse. Sex education is an area of increasing concern in national policy. Both the Department for Education and the Department of Health recognize the role of sex education as a key one in improving the nation's 'sexual health'. In particular *The Health of the Nation*, White Paper (DoH, 1992), has committed the government to take action aimed at reducing by half the number of unwanted teenage pregnancies by the year 2000. In addition, the government has identified sex education as important in the prevention of the spread of HIV/AIDS and other sexually transmitted diseases and also in terms of improving emotional and sexual relationships

(National Curriculum Council, 1990; DES, 1991; DfE, 1993; DoH, 1993). Sex education is, however, a hotly contested area, where perceptions of parental rights, 'best practice', the need to address sexual health and the rights of young people are almost continually in collision. The contested nature of sex education has resulted in confusion in official thinking, the Education Act 1993 providing the most recent example of this (see Redman 1994a and 1994b). The Act specifies: 1) that secondary schools and secondary pupils in special schools must be provided with sex education; 2) that sex education must include education about HIV and AIDS; and 3) that parents may withdraw pupils from sex education, except in so far as it falls within the statutory requirements of the National Curriculum. The Secretary of State is required, in this clause, to revise the National Curriculum so that science does not include HIV/AIDS, sexually transmitted diseases or 'aspects of human sexual behaviour other than biological aspects'.

While this topic area is not typical of health education in general, it has the useful function of constituting the extreme end of what teachers often consider their legitimate role to be, and it thus serves well to highlight a variety of ethical and professional issues that are often submerged in more general discussions of health education, though we believe these same issues also run under the surface of health education work on less contentious health topics such as nutrition and exercise.

We use as the principal vehicle for our thoughts in this chapter a study which elicited a range of concerns from a group of practising teachers who collaborated with us on a project designed to explore professional barriers to the introduction of effective education on sexual matters. The individual issues they raised are also picked up and examined in more detail with reference to the work of other commentators. In particular we examine the need for a review of the characteristics of the teaching-learning environment if health education is to be covered effectively. What are the implications for teaching style and classroom organization when the emphasis in the curriculum is on personal empowerment and the development of skills? Where does the teacher's responsibility for health education end, and how can teachers ensure that parents agree with the breadth of their intervention? How can school management systems support teachers in taking on this demanding role?

Between the devil and the deep blue sea: teachers talking

The study described here reports the work of a project undertaken with secondary school teachers and community workers in the Grampian region of Scotland as part of a broader research programme on the problems involved in educating young people about sexuality in general and about HIV/AIDS in particular.

Previous work with young people in focus groups and individual interviews (Hendry *et al.*, 1991) had revealed a classic picture of young people for the most part either denying that they had ever received any sex education or stating that what they had received was inappropriate and unhelpful, and this impression was compounded by interviews with a further set of young people as part of the preparation for the project reported here. Some programmes clearly still come from the Dark Ages of sex education. One interviewee, a girl in her late teens, remembering a lesson from school, opined:

> Sex education programmes should include ... everything about contraception ... not just the different types but how to use them. It should be about people, not sticklebacks.

On other occasions what passes as sex education is carried out in an atmosphere which is embarrassed, fraught and often chaotic. Girls frequently claim that boys in the classes disrupt any serious attempt to explore issues, and boys, while admitting their attempts to subvert such occasions, also resent it when girls are whisked away for separate tuition. One boy sums up:

> At school it was just funny ... ye either laugh or caper or slag it wi'

comments ... nae right discussion. We had a good teacher ... Mr McC and he would just yap and laugh with us ... he wasn't strict ... School stuff we knew by the time they got round to it and it was boring and a waste of time ... I don't think single sex groups are a good idea ... if it's all loons [boys] it's just muckin' aboot and arguments all the time. Quines [girls] tell ye tae shut up and ye do ...

Survey work in schools and community education settings had provided some further objective evidence of the patchiness and unsatisfactory nature of provision for sex education within the region, a finding confirmed by other authors (Scott and Thompson, 1992; Taylor and Brierley, 1992).

However the survey had also picked up deep-rooted concerns among education professionals who perceived the extent of the problem and the inadequacy of their offerings, but felt that remedying the deficit was beyond their capabilities. Interview follow-ups confirmed this impression and led to the establishment of the second short project which is reported here. The study was carried out in 1992 and set out to examine how young people's expectations about sex education compared with those of professional educators, and to explore the nature and extent of the problems facing professional educators in meeting those needs.

The heads of three secondary schools were approached and two agreed to take part in the study. The community education teams from the same catchments expressed interest and agreed to participate. The schools were selected for the contrast they presented in relation both to their catchment and to the approach which they had taken to developing sex education curricula. One catchment was centred around a community school with a planned approach to sex education implemented through a system of first-level guidance and a team interested in working together. The other was centred around a more traditional school just setting out to review its approach to sex education and with a team whose members had strongly differing perspectives on the topic.

At the beginning of the project a sample of young people outside these two catchments was recruited and interviewed individually about their experiences of sex education. The sample was recruited from hostels, youth groups, projects and training agencies. Two group discussions were held with young people in voluntary and statutory youth projects. Their perceptions and attitudes were then presented as a starting point to the sample of teachers and community workers who, over several months, worked alongside the research team, to explore a range of issues and to look at options for collaboration. The group met with research workers over four sessions and a workshop day. The content of the sessions was planned to explore 'neglected' areas and topics perceived as difficult to deal with for professionals engaged in sex education. The final workshop day was organized to examine some of the emerging themes with a broader range of professionals.

In-depth interviews were carried out with teachers in both catchments over several months after the initial fieldwork had been undertaken. The responses reported in this chapter relate principally to the teachers involved in the group. In reporting these we are heavily dependent on the fieldwork of Sieniewicz (1995).

Teachers and community workers identified a range of problems which confronted them as they attempted to respond to young people's need for better education on sex. Thus among both teachers and community educators there were problems identified about roles and interactions with individuals. These sit alongside concerns which relate more to problems within the institution in defining a curricular place for sex education and in the management of that role. Then too, there are broader issues concerning the extent to which educators (whether formal or informal) collaborate with or take into account the views of both parents and the wider community.

Concerns about professional identity and roles

It is a commonplace of sociological theory to view the school (and, by extension, the different forms of community education) as agents of secondary socialization in an era when the family has lost its potency as a major context for socializing young people for their adult roles (Jones and Wallace, 1992). One of the interests within the project was to ascertain the extent to which professional educators in both formal and informal settings had accepted this role as a reasonable part of their professional remit. To this end, one of the questionnaires described by Clift *et al.* (1989) was used to stimulate discussion in a workshop with teachers and community workers.

The discussion revealed no clear consensus, but rather a range of positions along a spectrum, even among a group whose enthusiasm and interest in the topic had caused them to volunteer for inclusion in the project. Interviews with a broader range of staff in both the case study schools confirmed these impressions.

Many teachers and community education workers were often happy enough to accept that they had a role to play by delivering straightforward information and statistics. They were happy to give young people information or addresses which would enable them to follow issues through on their own. They were not happy to talk about morality or relationships, or particularly about the nature of sexuality. Some people had adopted this role not out of a reluctance to confront the issues with young people (though this was clearly a feature for some) but because they resisted the notion that they were appropriate mentors in the realms of sex education. Some, for instance, were very conscious of the distance that their age created:

> There's another problem that I've got ... an age barrier. 'What does he know?' I'm in my fifties so 'what the hell does he know about this or that?'

But others characterized this problem not simply as one of age, but rather of length of time in the profession. In other words, those entering education twenty or thirty years ago held a different perspective on their professional role and responsibilities than did new entrants:

> In school and at college a few years ago it was made clear that

social education would be very much a part of what I was having to do at school. I haven't been teaching very long so what might seem like change to other teachers is just yet another new thing which is part of my teaching experience at the moment.

It is clear that age itself may simply be an intervening variable in determining one's professional identity, being a surrogate perhaps for confidence in one's own sexuality or one's ability to articulate issues around sex.

Many teachers and community educators saw their role going beyond the task of information-giving. Teachers talked about real learning only taking place where such facts were embedded in broader skills and they saw the sex education curriculum and their own role as being much more about the fostering of personal competencies and skills:

> I wouldn't be happy to just deliver information ... yes, some people would ... if the topic came round they'd be happy to deliver facts and figures without going too much into the morality and safety aspects.

> I think it's a responsibility to make sure that youngsters are aware of all the issues and their own attitudes ... that they get a chance to explore their attitudes and not necessarily just adopt attitudes from parents and the press.

Most interesting in some ways are those educators whose commitment to their charges and whose understanding of their role leads them into the realms of self-disclosure. One instinctively feels that it is only with these people that young people stand any chance of being able to explore the real dimensions of sexuality and sexual experience in addition to gaining information on the mechanics or the ethics of sex or being schooled in 'skills' they will need to negotiate their way through what is characterized as one of life's hazards:

> I have tried not to be inhibited in front of the kids. If they ask me a question ... unless it's really personal and they're only asking out of curiosity or to titillate the class ... I will answer truthfully, without compromising my professional status. They are curious and I don't really feel there is a whole area of my experience that I can block

97

them out of because it's so important for them to know things they haven't experienced. You have to give something of yourself. Giving of yourself brings out the relationship. Some teachers can only give information on subjects.

Among the self-disclosing teachers there was, however, a very real awareness of the risks of this strategy. Some of these rested in the difficulty of maintaining a professional persona within the school. Few felt that it threatened their ability to keep discipline or retain control, but many felt that there were awkward juxtapositions of their role as sex educators with that of their primary teaching role:

> You have to give something of yourself ... we're here with the pupils every day. It's difficult to give something of yourself but still keep the pupil's respect.
>
> Theoretically you shouldn't be a different teacher in science and social education, but in reality in science I will tell them to sit down, shut up and be quiet because I'm talking. In social education I'm a bit more flexible. We do have ground rules but they're more open.
>
> It's the role of the teacher within school that sets the remit ... they expect me to teach science ... 'what does he know about sex anyway?'

Many educators involved in the research project and also among the broader group subsequently interviewed had accepted their role as educators in this field and were prepared to put a lot of energy and thought into delivering education in an appropriate way. Despite playing the game like this, however, they still entertained doubts about the suitability of teachers as the prime agents in young peoples' sex education. Having a role as an authority figure, for instance, presents problems in taking on a remit for sex education, both for the teacher and for the pupil. Many teachers doubted their own ability to overcome the problem of young people seeing them as figures who police and evaluate them. One teacher commented on how he felt young people viewed them:

You might say something in the staff room or might write a report on them ... have it held against them.

And this was indeed backed up by comments from young people themselves.

Social class differences, age gaps and authority position were all factors cited by a number of teachers who wondered whether, with the best will in the world, they were the best people to act as mentors to young people in respect of sexual behaviour and attitudes:

> The kids don't necessarily identify with a teacher. We're middle class. We've got all these values which they regard often as being very moralistic ... which of course isn't necessarily true.

> They're quite right. That's how they react – quite literally. They don't say it, but I can see it. What do I know about 'E'? I don't know the peer pressure on them.

A young woman teacher in her early twenties noted:

> My tutor group asked 'How old are you when you stop having sex?' I said 'I don't know ... I can't remember.' It didn't get a laugh. They took the answer seriously!

Community education staff were less likely to voice this reservation. In part this was because their own educational experiences (particularly in the case of youth workers) had often been far from straightforward and they could use their own experience to relate to young people. Partly it was also due to a very different philosophy of working which de-emphasized the 'teacher' as the monopoly holder of knowledge and sought instead to work from young people's knowledge and understandings.

Rather more dangerous, many staff also felt, was the extent to which self-disclosing exchanges which had been appropriate in the context of lessons or group work in community settings might be taken out of context by others and used against them professionally. Teachers commented:

> I don't mind discussing my experiences and what I know ... From a

professional point of view it's a very dangerous area ... they might go home and tell their parents who might overreact ... might ring the school and then it might be my reputation or my entire career which is on the line.

If I start saying something like ... 'well, a few years ago I slept around a lot' ... they tell their parents. That's a danger. I'm not sure I should be saying that anyway.

One teacher commented knowingly on the extent to which the professional expectations of him by parents could be breached by someone in a different professional group. His comment is an interesting insight into the relative authority and status of different professional groups and the extent to which people will be prepared to use their power as parents to challenge the way in which their children are treated or services to their children are handled. Commenting on a visit by a local GP to a class of 12-year-olds which had resulted in an astonishing and outrageous performance by the doctor, he noted:

The whole issue of the status of the teacher ... he was using terminology ... words to shock the kids ... He knew what he was doing, but he has the status of a GP and I'm only a teacher. If I came out with this and the kids went home and said this, I'd be putting myself in a precarious position with the parents, the authorities and other bodies.

To summarize, teachers on the whole accept their role as 'agents of secondary socialization' within the specific context of education on sexuality, but interpretations of the extent of this role will vary from that of 'gatekeeper' through 'skill-developer' to 'discloser'. One might compare these with the different paradigms of health education discussed in the previous chapter. Even within the same school, and despite operating with the same course documents, teachers opt for a variety of modes of defining and addressing the problem. Moreover it is clear (though hardly surprising) that the majority of teachers do not see this as their prime professional role, given the structure of secondary education which prioritizes the academic disciplines within the curriculum in schools.

Among those who perceived this need to extend the role beyond that of merely being 'gatekeeper' to other sources of advice or help, there was, however, some doubt as to whether they were the most appropriate mentors of young people in this respect, even leaving aside the structural problems within the formal setting which problematized this role.

Teaching – learning issues

Curricular documents about health education in the 1970s and 1980s were, as we have noted in the previous chapter, considered to be in the vanguard of other developments in terms of the emphasis placed not so much on knowledge outcomes (though these were important), but also on the development of self-esteem and certain skills. What they have less to say about, however, is the learning skills and strategies that are involved in the acquisition and absorption of health education materials. Elias (1990) in making a case for health education, notes how important features of the learning context are for determining the success (or otherwise) of the experience:

> What this suggests is that instruction be given at least as much emphasis as curriculum because effective learning is unlikely to occur outside of children feeling engaged in the instructional process. This is not uniquely true of health education, but it is especially true of that field because the content and behaviours that are the focus are, ultimately, so personal and interpersonal in nature.
>
> (Elias, 1990, p.158)

He goes on to emphasize the importance of continuity and co-ordination in the curriculum (issues largely addressed now in the UK through the introduction of the 5 to 14 curriculum) but he also highlights the need for the curriculum to be flexible both in relation to new knowledge and also to the developmental needs of the children. Elias points at what we all know as parents and teachers, that 'children reach developmental milestones at somewhat different times' (Elias, 1990). A curriculum taught through large group didactic methods has little possibility of reacting flexibly to this situation.

101

Some authors have queried the salience of much school health education in respect of its failure to provide for the differential needs of boys and girls, for young people of ethnic minorities, and those whose sexual orientation does not conform to the heterosexist norm (Aggleton and Homans, 1988; Tones *et al.*, 1990). Tilford (1992) adds the group of young people with disabilities to this list, and also notes how few schools have developed health education policies 'which have strongly and clearly addressed inequalities in health' (Tilford, 1992).

A further 'common denominator' noted by Elias (1990) that needs to be incorporated into health education programmes is that of 'engagement'. Noting that health education is only a very small part of the school, social and family activities in which most adolescents engage, he comments wryly that:

> Clearly, educators cannot assume that the subject matter has so much intrinsic appeal that students will put aside other concerns and fully absorb what is presented to them.　(Elias, 1990, p.159)

It is in relation to this notion of 'engagement' that we draw most closely towards the actual classroom processes and the relationship between pupil and teacher. Elias characterizes the processes variously known as constructive engagement, respectful engagement or dialoguing as:

> active respectful listening, open-ended questioning which stimulates representational thinking and reflection about affect and behaviour, reciprocal sharing, a climate of acceptance, and a commitment to fostering the self-regulation of children.
>
> (Elias, 1990, p.161)

Such an approach is thus essentially pupil-centred, highlights skill development, but is also ostensibly about encouraging pupils to make contributions from their own experience and about adopting a posture which does not criticize practices or behaviours which may be different or dangerous or illegal (Arborelius and Bremberg, 1988).

In practice there is cause for doubt that many schools find this an easy or a practical model to operate. Coggans *et al.*

(1991a) in a review of drugs education programmes comment:

> In the case of school-based drug education the reality is that the extent to which the pupil-centred approach is followed will be constrained by teachers' concerns about the illegality of drugs and the attitudes of society at large towards drugs. Accordingly, descriptions of drug education approaches as 'life skills', 'decision-making skills' are disingenuous to the extent that the decision has already been made for the pupil. (Coggans *et al.*, 1991a, p.1108)

Elsewhere these same authors (1991b) note the difficulty of 'selling' a decision-making approach to schoolchildren on health issues within the context of a school which allows no consultation, participation or decision-making in relation to other aspects of school life. Their recipe for change reinforces the notion that health education programmes must be based within a whole-school context, but this notion is infinitely more challenging than that usually understood by the health-promoting school. For many schools the adoption of healthy tuck-shops and canteens or no-smoking zones in staff rooms is radical enough. The idea that staff should really allow young people to make their own decisions, even if these ran counter to the knowledge and mores of the teacher is very difficult.

The less charitable might see in this merely the reluctance of benevolent autocrats to cede power or to admit that they don't always know best. Many teachers, however, feel a real professional dilemma about the extent to which they are *in loco parentis*. If they know a child is behaving dangerously or in a way prejudicial to their well-being they are often torn between their duty to parents (or as proxy parents) and their duty to respect and accept young people's confidences. This is never an easy dilemma to resolve.

Beyond this, teaching staff face another dilemma in relation to values and norms in health education. Many of the values expressed by children are, for instance, heavily gendered and/or homophobic. Some of the comments by young people interviewed as part of the study described in the previous section illustrate this point graphically:

There are three Fs when you spik aboot women ... fancy them, fuck them and forget them.

Same sex ... it just makes me take a temper. The first poofter I ever met was JoJo in second year. He said he was gonnae rape me. Ever since ... hate them. If ye sit wi' the craws ye get shot wi' them.

Many educationalists would see it as a very positive part of their role to challenge these 'negative' values, yet this sits rather uneasily with Coggans *et al.*'s (1991a and 1991b) notion that young people's views must be accepted and used as a starting point.

Moreover different aspects of health promotional work offer up conflicting and paradoxical messages to staff and students alike. We are, for instance, to be told very clearly what's good for us in terms of diet and exercise. There is no tiptoeing around on this – health promotion experts know what's best for us, they'll tell us and we are supposed to oblige by behaving rationally. In relation to sex or drugs, however, the new message is that while the experts might know what's good for us, they realize that they must accept existing behaviours and work with those without passing judgement. Such conflicts in the ethos of health education as it is currently taught do little to improve confidence in teachers or trust in pupils.

Other authors have interpreted the value of health (and knowledge about health) as being related to these issues of locus of control and autonomy. Massey (1990) notes that health education in schools has chiefly subscribed to this empowerment model – indeed, it is enshrined in some of the earliest curricular documents looked at in the previous chapter.

However, as we have seen, concepts of autonomy can be interpreted negatively as a political tool to deny the structural social and economic forces which confine us within certain lifestyles. French and Adams explore the relationship between these approaches, suggesting that there is an overlap:

the acceptance that generally to be healthy and educated leads to increasing degrees of autonomy and to be unhealthy and uneducated leads to decreasing autonomy, and consequently loss of power and control over one's health status. (French and Adams, 1986, p.72)

It is clear then that health education is a contested concept.

The generation of 'voice': collaboration with parents

One of the classic features involved in teachers' fears of embarking upon more sustained work on issues of sexuality is their claim that they cannot be sure of the extent to which educational stakeholders (in particular parents) desire them to do this and will support them in the endeavour.

A considerable volume of empirical work exists demonstrating that, on the whole, parents are happy to entrust schools with education around sexual issues (Allen, 1987). In fact they may be more than willing to share their parental responsibilities or even offload them on to educators because of their own sense of inadequacy for the task (Farquhar, 1990; Frankham *et al.*, 1992).

The literature on adolescence suggests that parents continue to have influence over significant aspects of adolescents' lives. However we know little of the models of knowledge, lay beliefs or values which parents operate. There is also a gap in our knowledge of how young people themselves interpret and make use of the advice and information gleaned from the home (Brannen *et al.*, 1994).

An interview study with young people reported by Hendry *et al.* (1991) showed that, for a number of respondents, parental trust in their children was seen as important for enabling discussion to take place. Where this did not happen, young people viewed parents as having little to contribute. In relation to sexual matters, many felt education was better carried out away from the home, since it was too difficult for both parents and children to tackle such topics without embarrassment:

> I think my generation is less closed than my parents. We have been
> exposed to more things. Different ways of treating sex and that it
> can be talked about. Their embarrassment is hard to take, especially
> if you're not sure.   (Girl, rural, in Hendry *et al.*, 1991b, p.15)

Within many families the topic of sex education has highly
emotional overtones and can be shrouded in mystery and
uncertainty especially when children reach adolescence. Some
adolescents express reluctance to discuss sexually related
matters with their parents although some evidence indicates
that attitudes and beliefs derive from informal talk in the home
especially with mothers (Hendry *et al.*, 1993b; Allen, 1987;
Wyness, 1991).

West (1993) has characterized the extent to which schools
give clear statements about their value systems and consult
with parents and others about the negotiation of these values
as an issue of 'voice', following on from the earlier work of
Hirschman (1970).

Few schools have the courage to develop 'voice' or to engage
in real dialogue with their community in relation to such
contentious issues as sex education. Some may take soundings
from random contacts with parents. Others may take parental
quiescence as a sign of approval. A common strategy, for
example, in schools, is to send a brief note to parents at the
start of a term in which some particular input on sexual
matters is to be tackled. Parents will be told about the happening and asked to contact school if they have any queries, but
rarely is detail entered into concerning the school's viewpoint
on homosexuality, the provision of contraceptive information
to under 16s and so on:

> You write an open letter and say if they object do so in writing and
> that pupil will be removed from the group. And if they do not reply
> you assume that that is tacit agreement to go on with it.

It would be a brave school which undertook an exercise with
parents to explore what input they felt they and their children
'needed' or whether it was possible to reach a consensual position on contentious issues:

Parents may not react in the same way to a question such as 'Do you want your child to operate out of ignorance?' as they would to 'Do you want your child to be told about anal sex and mainlining?'

Interviews with teachers explored this theme of developing a dialogue with parents which would strengthen their professional position and enhance the effectiveness of what they offered to pupils. For most teachers the option is not one they can undertake officially without the sanction of senior management, and few felt sanguine about getting approval from a management team which felt it was better to let sleeping dogs lie. The rhetoric from a member of the senior management team in one of the case study schools sounded encouraging:

> I think if you get parents in and you explain what you're about to parents ... have a communication with parents, then you can take parents with you. Certainly you can take the majority of the parents with you.

But as a teacher from the same school glumly noted:

> We've always thought we should have a night when we have the parents in but it's difficult to get parents in. When we did Skillseekers (about careers) only a couple of parents turned up that night, so I don't think we'd get a lot ... We talked about it, but we've never done it ... the headmaster ... some sensitive stuff in the video ... but we've never done it. We'd like parents to see it.

Perhaps there is some justification for this reluctance. Arkin (1993) for instance reports on a project undertaken in Birmingham to enhance the way in which schools market meetings with parents. Attendance is notoriously poor at secondary level, particularly among that sector of parents with which one might wish to engage most actively. The report highlights the difficulties encountered, commenting on 'the tradition of education in which parents, preoccupied with their own children, are content to leave the running of schools to 'the professionals'. Arkin's short article highlights the need for schools not to be defeatist about this but to look at the examples of good practice being developed by some schools and in community education.

In the realm of sex education there is even more reason to suppose that attendance at such events by parents might not be welcomed by young people themselves. Many of the letters of invitation might never make it home and out of the school bag for fear that parents might want to raise big issues about it at home:

> Lots of parents don't know what is going on anyway, because kids don't release this information to parents because of their own embarrassment. Parents don't actually know that there are no clear guidelines. Maybe that haziness in the middle is a protection for both parties at the end of the day.

The dangers inherent in a more democratic and participatory model of educational practice are not lost on teachers since the introduction of school boards. Participation or the development of 'voice' is too often restricted to those parents better equipped to represent their views or to those with a particularly strong hobby-horse or lobby, and the mechanisms in place in relation to this participation do not protect the rights of the silent majority from a vociferous but small contingent with unrepresentative but strongly held views:

> There are some parents who are very vociferous, and I think if it was them that complained ... your chances of getting backed would be less than if it wasn't.

Hirschman's analysis (1970) of the way in which market forces might impact on education saw the obvious mechanism by which such markets would operate as that of 'exit'. In other words, parents acting on behalf of their children would vote with their feet and change schools once legislation was put in place which allowed them the freedom to choose and the information with which to make that choice. Education in Scotland in the last ten years has seen those mechanisms put in place in the form of parental right of choice, the publication of school prospectus information and league tables of performance indicators. As West (1993) notes, the obvious reaction (though not the best in her opinion) is for heads to act strategically but defensively to limit exit. They might do this by nurturing very carefully the image of the school, bolstering the positive and playing down the negative. In these circumstances it is not hard to see why heads might shy away from any controversy around the school's sex education policy:

> The head is in the business of selling the school ... he wants the school to have a good reputation in the area ... he wants parents to think every thing here is fine, because otherwise parents have the choice to send their children elsewhere.

> I think the head would not want to make a great thing of this. I think he would feel happier if there were strong regional guidelines – and a definite regional policy – because he could then say to parents 'Look ... the region says it's important to deal with this ... contraception, homosexuality' ... He feels an element of vulnerability. If the school was criticized by certain groups of parents ... and publicized ... then he would get no backing from the region ...

A similar point is made by Coffield and Gofton (1994), who note a further dimension of the dilemma facing teachers who wish to pursue a realistic drug education programme. The new market-driven situation in education in which schools compete for pupils and, ultimately, resources, means that many head teachers are loath to accept that there is a drug problem in the locality and that they should raise the profile of the issue through a comprehensive education programme:

> In other words, the Government's educational strategy is placing structural constraints in the way of teachers who wish to introduce drug education. Because of the operations of the free market, there is now less space than ever before for the open discussion of controversial issues.   (Coffield and Goften, 1994, p.32)

Teachers also comment on their reluctance to assume that the values they hold are consonant with that of adults generally in the catchment within which they teach. Should they be acting *in loco parentis* in delivering information, advice or developing skills with which parents would happily identify, or should they operate within an agenda which is more professional, probably more 'politically correct' and profoundly more middle class?

> The barriers exist due to their upbringing. They are confronted by things my imagination can hardly take in. It's completely foreign to me ... so different. The number of pupils here confronted by changing fathers, changing everything ... it's so different. And I've raised a barrier there. I now realize that that does go on. Until I came to this area I didn't. The whole sense of values is different.

Children, too, find themselves caught between the norms promoted by the school, which parents too may pay lip service to, and the reality of life as it is lived in their community. Hendry *et al.* (1991) report the following comment from a teenage girl:

> Your father says don't smoke when he has a cigarette in his hand and don't drink when the following weekend he's out at the bar getting drunk. (Girl S2, suburbs, Hendry *et al.*, 1991, p.24)

Recent attempts in Scotland to improve school effectiveness highlight the need for schools to explore their ethos, and packages issued by the Scottish Office Education Department encourage schools to audit feelings among their staff, their pupils and their parent group, at first by means of simple questionnaires supplied in the package. Though these refer nowhere to specific curricular issues, and certainly not to sex education, the point is made that schools can no longer afford to operate in this isolated and aloof way from the communities that they serve if they are to be seen as 'effective schools'.

The foregoing discussion ignores the 'voice' issue which teachers and community workers mention frequently, namely that of developing and sustaining a dialogue with young people themselves about their needs in relation to sex education. We have referred to this, however, in Chapter 3.

Managing health education in schools: support or mediation?

The two case study schools in our study presented marked contrasts in the way in which sex education was handled managerially. The seemingly more progressive and 'thought out' school with its policy of first level guidance had a clear curriculum and good materials, a supportive guidance team, friends in the senior management team who made all the right noises. In reality the first level guidance system dragooned into the sex education programme a range of teachers. Many staff felt ill-equipped personally to undertake teaching of the kind that was clearly required by the set materials and resented the sense in which they had been dragged into delivering lessons with what they knew was not the right approach to the topic:

> It is such a personal thing it can become ... y'know ... I think it can be threatening. I don't think you can expect people unless they feel comfortable to be a lot more than deliverers of information ... I don't know if they've got the right to say they won't do it, but they've got the right to say 'this is as far as I want to go' ...

In reality the option of staying uncommitted because you feel inadequately prepared for the task is not always there in some schools. A senior member of the management team in this same school who claimed he did not believe in coercion management nevertheless stated:

> when we interview them for the school we make sure we ask them to take a part in the extracurricular regime of the school – the tutorial programme – if it comes down to the wire, they have agreed.

In contrast the more traditional school had accepted that not all teachers felt able or willing to teach sex education in an appropriate way and, while offering training and support, had not coerced the reluctant into participation.

Some thoughts in conclusion

What then might we say in summary about the difficulties imposed by professional identity and the difficulty of developing partnership or dialogue with parents on this topic?

Firstly, that these issues of professional identity and voice are strongly linked. The former seems to provide a number of barriers to school work on sex education which will probably only be overcome by the development of a new professionalism which does not shirk the expression of its values and which seeks out the views of its catchment in just the way advocated by West (1993).

Secondly, that schools must work harder at the development of a consensus about the appropriateness of involvement on these issues. Simply assuming consensus is not enough as it will result in widely differing qualities of engagement and presentation even where a programme has been standardized.

Thirdly, that all education professionals require appropriate support if they are to tackle such contentious and demanding work with young people. Training and resources help, but they are not enough. Teachers need to know that there are clear guidelines for their operation, and that while they stay within these guidelines they will receive full managerial support to protect their personal and professional standing.

Fourthly, that schools and their pupils gain little by adopting programmes which involve teachers who lack confidence and training to tackle sex-related issues.

Fifthly, that the development of 'voice' with parents is a difficult but necessary part of the professional role, if education professionals are to deliver a curriculum on these issues which is appropriate and which has the backing of parents. Such an attempt requires innovative ways of making contact with and developing dialogue in a way that ensures that all views are heard and listened to.

5 Educating in the community

Introduction

We have seen in previous chapters how traditional approaches to educational work with young people on health have met with limited success. It is clear that some groups of young people have rejected or are themselves marginalized by classic or formal approaches to health education. Findings from empirical research suggest that some youth populations have proved persistently difficult to access.

In general, it could be argued that the lack of a coherent theoretical framework for health education which takes account of the diversity and changing experiences of youth inhibits the development of more appropriate interventions.

In this chapter the role of community-based education on health with young people will be explored as providing a possible avenue for taking account of the varying perspectives of young people. In particular the relevance of community development approaches will be examined in relation to the aims of health promotion and youth work. Discussion of how these can be reconciled in developing frameworks for educational work with young people on health concerns will follow.

Taking account of diversity

In this chapter we explore how health education interventions remain heavily based on promoting individual change. This is in the face of evidence from a range of research studies and evaluations over a number of years suggesting the need to consider the impact of structural constraints (Coffield and Gofton, 1994; Aggleton 1989). In addition, young people themselves have provided a wealth of accounts in research studies, TV documentaries and other media reports which challenge this focus in their criticisms of the style and content of offerings available to them (Hendry *et al.*, 1991).

Such strategies of individual empowerment fail to take account of the structural inequalities faced by different groups of young people. For example young homeless people may attach a low priority to health matters until they can resolve more pressing practical issues in their lives (Kirk *et al.*, 1991; Shelter, 1993; Fisher and Collins, 1993). The contradictory sets of expectations placed on young women in managing their reputation often means that adopting health messages will be a risky process (Holland *et al.*, 1990a and 1990b). Studies have also shown that young men face tensions between maintaining an image of having knowledge and experience on sexual matters, while at the same time having fears of failing to live up to this image (Wight, 1993; Holland *et al.*, 1993). The literature is also peppered with expressions of fear by young people that sex education may reveal gay or bisexual identities (Holland *et al.*, 1993; Bell, 1991). Many classic health education approaches also fail to recognize the importance of cultural difference and diversity. Thus forms of intervention based on individualistic models tend to decontextualize health education to the extent that it becomes irrelevant or dissonant with young people's own experience.

It is clear then, that at both theoretical and empirical levels there is a need to address the range of cultural, social and political contexts within which young people in the UK are managing the transition to adulthood. Many of the issues facing young people are interlinkings of concerns about self-identity, relationships with family, peers and friends on the one hand and structural constraints such as unemployment, culture, housing and poverty on the other (Coffield *et al.*, 1986). Thus young people in adolescence are presented with challenges which have highly significant social dimensions. In the past it is true to say that much research relating to health education needs and receptivity has focused on the maturational psychological aspects of young people's lives at the expense of these social and cultural dimensions. More recently, concern about the spread of HIV has resulted in a sharper focus on cultural aspects of knowledge and belief, and so has examined, for instance, how young people themselves perceive and interpret themes of sexuality and risk (Woodcock *et al.*, 1992; Hendry *et al.*, 1991).

In turn this highlights the necessity to adopt educational methods which stimulate and enhance participation and take account of the themes of control and trust which have been noted as lacking in many interventions aimed at young people on health matters. To compound the challenge this transformation has to take place within a climate of confusion at governmental, national and local level as witnessed in debates about the place and scope of sex education (Scott and Thompson, 1992). In this respect, the role of the media in setting the agenda cannot be overemphasized.

Given the heterogeneity of young people's experience and the variety of conditions which structure their behaviour and beliefs is there reason to believe that informally based learning which starts from and works with young people's own perspectives offers more hope of success? We firstly investigate how strategies based on self-empowerment models offer a more promising move towards a recognition of the complexities facing young people. However this promise is not fulfilled since there is little genuine recognition of the structural contexts within which young people operate. We go on to explore some dimensions of community and investigate the potential of strategies based on community development principles. Despite some caveats, we argue that this may offer a genuine alternative.

Empowerment-based strategies

In response to the demand for more person-centred approaches, there have been considerable attempts to promote skills-based packages on health education. These stress the need to develop decision-making skills, assertiveness and the ability to negotiate. Major themes are empowerment and self-efficacy. In research terms, the health belief and health action models discussed in Chapter 3 have been influential. Ingham *et al.* (1992) succinctly summarize how research effort should be redirected in this direction.

> New theoretical approaches to understanding health related behaviour require a shift away from an obsession with individual knowledge or attitude scores on questionnaires towards the elucidation of meanings, powers, liabilities and constraints, from simple concepts of illness avoidance towards an acknowledgement of the importance of social reputations and from crude frequencies towards the dynamic processes involved in creating and maintaining identities. (Ingham *et al.*, 1992, p.171)

Methods aimed at increasing self-empowerment have been devised and used by educators both in formal and informal settings (see Shucksmith *et al.*, 1993, for a recent review). Such initiatives have sprung from a recognition of the need to develop some understanding of young people's own perspectives and lay beliefs as starting points for interventions which are seen as more relevant and ultimately more acceptable to young people themselves.

However, many of these approaches still remain firmly based on encouraging individual change with little cognizance taken of the structural context within which young people operate. The fostering of assertiveness and negotiation skills which are the fare of this approach may be worthwhile in building confidence but have little impact or, worse, may be positively undermining if the person to be negotiated with is reluctant to co-operate or to negotiate at all. For young women especially this can pose risks in both physical and emotional terms in the absence of understanding of the situations within which such negotiations may take place. A clichéd, but nevertheless apt, example of this, is how young women who are known to carry condoms are perceived to be promiscuous by both other women and men, which carried a number of implications for them.

Friendship, peers and community

Young people's friendship groups are frequently assumed to be the opponent of the health educator in the educational scenario, encouraging subversive behaviour and providing a counter to attempts to instil healthy practices. With this perspective, little recognition is made of the shifting nature of power within groups and of the dynamic nature of interactions within and between different groups of peers. The notion of peer education challenges this view, aiming to build on the positive aspects of peer relationships, as Pearson (1987) indicates in discussing the friendship patterns of young drug users:

> It would be wrong to think of these contexts of friendship as only concerning 'bad company' which can lead people astray. Friendship can be both the route into certain kinds of drug choices and the way out. And even within a single friendship network, different people will nevertheless exercise different options and at different times, in such a way that the outcomes of their heroin experiences will significantly differ.   (Pearson, 1987, p.84)

Peer education attempts to bring peer groups into the health education arena by working with rather than against them. However under the umbrella of the label of peer education a range of different perspectives have been identified, some of which rely heavily on notions of self-empowerment. These issues are explored more fully in the following chapter.

Changing patterns of behaviour and especially lifestyle are frequently cited as a goal of health education (Bellingham and Gillies, 1993). Thus little attention is paid to the reasons and meanings which young people themselves give for adopting certain forms of behaviour. It is assumed that young people will respond more positively to repackaging of the messages rather than a complete redesign! Consequently the victim-blaming which has characterized classic approaches to health education can be reinforced. Interventions which are covert 'decision implementation' models in the guise of decision-making models have been roundly criticized as ineffective in a recent evaluation of drugs education in schools (Coggans *et al.*, 1990).

The reluctance among educators to focus on the social dimensions rather than the individual has been noted in a number of commentaries. As Blaxter concludes in a recent study of lifestyles and health:

> Education aimed at the personal modification of lifestyles may be resisted if the power to change is, or is felt to be, unavailable. The ability to choose is inevitably restricted by living and working conditions. (Blaxter, 1990, p.243)

Nevertheless it cannot be denied that education has a vital role to play in helping young people to manage the changes in moving towards adulthood, however ill-defined this adult status might be. Community development may offer some insight into approaches which take account of some of the difficulties outlined in this section.

Community development

Community development is a term which has increasing currency in the language of health promotion: the widely cited World Health Organization definition of health promotion specifically refers to community development as a mechanism for helping meet the needs of the whole population:

> The growth of health promotion has been built on public rather than medical-professional interest. It is linked to a growing interest in the general public in positive health, in personal growth and in community development. (WHO, 1982, p.3)

Health promotion thus explicitly recognizes that social, political and economic factors are influences on health behaviour and in so doing, recognizes the limitations of traditional health education.

Community participation and education on health

The term community has widespread appeal and this has been demonstrated by the current fashion of tacking 'community' on to a range of professional disciplines or jobs e.g. the Care in the Community motif. Mayo (1991) refers to the plethora of definitions of community and the wide range of assumptions about the meaning of the term. However it is important to differentiate between rhetorical use of the notion and the actual processes of community development, education and participation.

Community education refers to a profession or para-profession within which community development approaches inform how the worker identifies, works with and relates to the community. Such workers have an explicitly educational role, but they have no statutory educational remit. They may work alongside or outwith formal settings such as schools. Commonly community education workers have a remit to carry out youth work, adult education and community development. Similarly community workers may be employed by voluntary agencies or local authorities to work mainly in neighbourhoods around locally identified issues. Community workers may also adopt community development strategies as part of their practice. The Federation of Community Work Training Groups training manual gives a recent definition of community work which specifically includes health within the range of issues to be addressed (FCWTG, 1993).

The idea of community development has been around for a long time, particularly in the fields of community education and youth work where it has had a particular role in work with powerless or marginalized groups. With its roots in colonialism it was re-imported to the West where it was adopted in attempts to regenerate declining inner cities especially in the early 1970s. Its influence was clear in both the American War on Poverty Headstart programmes and the British community development projects. Community development is a major element of development strategies in developing countries in Africa and South America (Dudley, 1993).

119

The Association of Metropolitan Authorities used a community development perspective to examine the key issues facing local government in exploring their role in the 1990s seeing this perspective as a means of recognizing the cultural diversity within and building working partnerships with and between the communities which they serve (AMA, 1993). There are many different models of community development and there is no intention here to rework these but rather to highlight those aspects which may be particularly relevant to debates around young people and health. For the purposes of this discussion community development will be investigated as a strategy, rather than an aim, as this permits us to see it as being relevant to a diversity of professional groups as well as having the potential to foster mutual understanding between and within these groups. Moreover, examined in this way, the usefulness of the approach for educators working with different groups of young people can be highlighted. Themes of empowerment, control and learning through organization are central to the concept. The theoretical framework has been heavily influenced by the writings and work of Paulo Freire (1972).

Freire developed his theory of 'conscientization' as a basic means of effecting social change, building up from dialogue between those who are disenfranchised and using group work in 'culture circles' as the mechanism for exploring issues, identifying problems and finding ways in which these can be tackled. Through this process, both the subjective understandings and the structural contexts of individual lives are uncovered. Groups can then identify means of dealing with the problem, using both their own experience and appropriate expertise. The processes of action and reflection are important themes which are continually revisited. Education is about building on experience, making sense of that experience and using technical assistance as required. This technical assistance may take a variety of forms, depending on the nature of the problem and proposed solutions.

Education is thus identified as a liberating process in which people are the subjects of their own learning. For Freire the process of education is never neutral and must serve as a means of liberating the oppressed. The role of the educator is to work with the group rather than to impose a curriculum or set of ideas. Descriptions such as 'animateur' and 'facilitator' suggest the process is collaborative and one of posing problems together, reflecting on these through dialogue, and uncovering the underlying issues. Professional expertise is called on to help solve a problem rather than to set the agenda. Thus the experience lying within the community is recognized and forms the basis for action, while the abilities of those living in difficult circumstances are recognized rather than problematized. Freire describes this as cultural synthesis, contrasting it with imposed or 'top down' forms of education which he calls the 'banking' system of education. With the 'banking' system educators practice 'cultural invasion' uncritically drawing on their own values and ideology. In contrast 'cultural synthesis' he describes as a process whereby the educators come to learn about the world and the themes of participants in a climate of mutual respect (Freire, 1972).

It is argued that through participating in group activity, key issues can be identified and learning will take place through a partnership with educators. Learning takes place at individual and collective level, being first and foremost the development of critical skills, based on the sharing of experience and the development of strategies for change at both personal and political levels.

Although Freire's work was undertaken in South America, his influence has been substantial in the development of initiatives in community settings in Western Europe, the USA and developing countries in Africa. His stance that education is not neutral but should involve both critical thinking and action to enable people to take control over their lives and transform their reality has implications at individual, collective and societal levels.

Is there a community of youth?

In this section we will look at ideas of community which are relevant to young people and explore how these have the potential for an examination of the idea of a community of youth.

The notion of community is frequently related to neighbourhood and geographical contexts as Tones *et al.* (1990) outline:

> A community is distinguished from any other social aggregation in respect of its relative size, geographical contiguity and the nature of the social network and norms prevailing within this circumscribed locality. (Tones *et al.*, 1990, p.235)

However there have been significant changes in understandings of community. This has come about for a variety of reasons, not least the interest and scrutiny community development has been subjected to in recent years. Better understanding of the role of race and gender have also informed current attempts to define community development (FCWTG, 1992). The notion of communities of interest has also gained currency and provides a particularly useful framework for exploring the potential for health promotion in relation to young people. Two kinds of development which highlight specific aspects of community development processes will be briefly examined in the section which follows.

There has been a significant increase in the range of women's community health initiatives over the last twenty years. Although many of these initiatives begin with a locality orientation, many have tackled health issues in ways which owe little to the notion of geographical neighbourhood. The development of a strategy arises from discussion and debate, linking private and public concerns and with an explicitly educational approach. The structure of these organizations is seen as important in encouraging involvement at a range of levels and most aim to operate on an individual and group basis (Jones and Graham, 1992; Orr, 1987).

Such groups have often organized around holistic definitions of health which challenge the notion that medical experts hold a monopoly on health knowledge. To this end, the educational content is based on the premise that women themselves have important experience and knowledge which they can

122

share both within the group, with other women and with medical professionals whose specialized knowledge is thus placed within the wider context. Personal development is only one aspect of this process, with some groups developing self-help initiatives within an area to enable discussion and to provide support for other women. Many groups have also been influential in campaigns for changes in policies and practices at both local and national levels while their critiques of health services have, in some cases, informed the development of new initiatives such as the establishment of Well Woman services within GP clinics locally or the challenging of prescribing patterns of benzo-diazepanes nationally. Some projects explicitly draw on the philosophy and practice of Freire as well as on feminist theories of gender and inequality (Kirkwood and Kirkwood, 1989).

In a similar way, the development of a range of voluntary and action groups within gay communities in the light of the HIV/AIDS crisis has challenged orthodoxies about gay experience (Aggleton *et al.*, 1993). Many of these organizations, such as the Terrence Higgins Trust, Scottish Aids Monitor and Outrage, have developed educational strategies not only for the gay community but for the wider population, seeing their role as challenging homophobia in both public and private spheres (Altman, 1993). Clearly not all men who have sex with men identify themselves as part of a gay community, nor do all gay men form one homogeneous group. But it is clear that within some gay communities, many have accepted safer sex messages. Despite concern about the realities of sustaining these educational 'gains' among some groups, nevertheless this seems to be one of the few populations where rates of HIV infection have been lowered by dynamic, well-targeted and acceptable health education (Johnson *et al.*, 1994; Dowsett *et al.*, 1992).

Ownership of the issue has been central to these developments, which arose out of anger at the neglect by medics, other professionals and policy-makers of HIV/AIDS issues when it was assumed to be a so called 'gay disease' (Shilts, 1988). Gay

123

men perceived themselves to be powerless in the face of the crisis unless they organized to resist dominant homophobic policies and practices. Watney argues that many of the gay health education initiatives have aimed to correct misapprehensions and myths, some of which have found their way into early health education campaigns about HIV/AIDS (Watney, 1993).

In relation to the same issue, consciousness-raising has been a feature of many educational initiatives, demonstrations and lobbies of parliament both within gay settings and in policy-making arenas, with one of the most successful examples being the Stonewall campaign around the lowering of the gay male age of consent in 1994. A major theme has been to redefine ideas about sexuality at a community level, encouraging gay and lesbian pride in their community and the development of safer sex as a means of safeguarding not only the existence of this community but challenging dominant attitudes to sexuality and gender. Clearly, however, to assume there is one gay community is to minimize the heterogeneity and diversity of gay culture and to underestimate the range of different groups with their own specific concerns. Frankenberg's (1966) notion of community seems, however, to contain within it a recognition of such diversity and the ways in which it is accommodated:

> Community implies having something in common ... Their common interest in things give them a common interest in each other. They quarrel with each other but are never indifferent to each other. They form a group of people who meet frequently face to face although this may mean they end up back to back. That people in such an area of social life turn their backs on each other is not a matter of chance. In a community even conflict may be a form of co-operation. (Frankenberg, 1966, p.238)

Johnson *et al.* (1994) have noted that it is only within the gay movement and the women's press, for example, that the promotion of safer sex (other than condom use or reduction in numbers of partners) has been prominent. In this sense community development has been 'transformatory', in

Aggleton's terms, in attempting to challenge dominant sets of beliefs and practices which marginalize particular groups (Aggleton *et al.*, 1993).

Targeting young gay men with health education has been a major focus of these campaigns and this highlights the absence of such education in schools. Indeed research findings confirm the silence on the topic of homosexuality within school settings.

Assessing young people's knowledge and perceptions

Until recently, most research into adolescents and health was undertaken in schools often for no other reason than the purely pragmatic one that it was here that the widest cross-section of young people could be contacted relatively easily and persuaded to participate. Undoubtedly the findings of such studies have contributed vital knowledge and enhanced understanding of many aspects of young people's needs and aspirations. Moreover, much of the data can be compared across regions, countries and cultures.

However it is also clear that school settings may not be appropriate settings for some forms of research study. For some young people the school setting may be a site of conflict and alienation especially in relation to health-related topics: those who perceive a need to disguise emerging sexual identities, for example, or to suppress information on social circumstances and family arrangements may find the mere presence of research studies can amplify risks and expose them to ridicule or harassment. For example, some young gay men interviewed in a study carried out by the authors were unanimous in declaring that school was something to survive without giving away any clues about their sexuality, even where this meant colluding with anti-gay views (Hendry *et al.*, 1991). For this group, the introduction of single-sex groups for health education was seen as posing risks since it would be more likely to demand greater participation and discussion which might lead to disclosure or challenge.

Existing drug users also had a realistic understanding of the dangers of being identified and this, for some, demanded a high level of discretion within school. Examples of exclusions and expulsions of known drug users were frequently cited in discussions with young people. A number of students simply opt out of attending school to a greater or lesser extent, and official statistics are limited in their ability to reflect the diversity of truancy patterns. Some may sign in at the first period and then leave for the day. Others may quietly disappear for weeks at a time. Some young people devise sophisticated tactics for staying away without appearing in official statistics of truancy. In other instances young people may resist by refusing to engage with school and, by extension, any research based there.

In some settings parents may use their right to withdraw their children from taking part in any research studies. Furthermore some schools may be constrained by their own structures to limit access to research into sensitive areas where questions over prevalence of drug-taking activity, availability of drugs within an area, levels of sexual activity and so on may be sought. In the current climate of competition for students, some heads are reluctant to allow exploration of any such topic fearing the reputation of the school may be jeopardized.

We labour this point perhaps merely to highlight the issue that many classic studies of young people, because of settings in which they were undertaken, probably overemphasize the homogeneity of the youth experience and may, in effect, be sanitized or impoverished by the perception held by the researcher of the young person in school. Thus it may be more appropriate to undertake such research in settings where young people feel comfortable and where diversity is accepted rather than problematized. However this raises some interesting methodological and sampling questions which demand creative responses. For example finding such young people out of school settings may be a costly and time-consuming process. Inevitably such a strategy will result in smaller and more localized samples with which sustained contact may also be problematic. Some researchers have succeeded in developing strategies whereby they recruit through schools but then transport participants out of school to more informal settings (Coffield and Gofton, 1994). Some of these methodological questions will be considered below. Firstly however it is important to identify the sort of groups which may be absent from existing studies.

To this end it may be useful to explore briefly some of the gaps in the literature on youth and health to pinpoint more accurately just who is likely to be absent. The impact of government policy changes in relation to education, social security and housing in particular have had a powerful impact on young people (Jones and Wallace, 1992; Hollands, 1990). For example it is clear that the number of homeless young people is on the increase in most areas of the UK. It is also increasingly clear that these numbers are largely made up of those who have few traditional forms of support, having been in care, custody or mental hospitals (Kirk *et al.*, 1991). In addition, many young people are more dependent on their parents now than in the last twenty years. The role of health and perceptions of its importance in young people's lives must be viewed within this changing political, economic and social context.

The invisibility of young women is a recurring theme in much feminist analysis of youth (McRobbie, 1991; Deem, 1989). Marshall and Borrill (1984) highlight some of the problems they found in making contact with young women in youth work settings in a study undertaken in the North of England:

> The problems we encountered in contacting young women made us appreciate why so much research has been done with all male groups and with captive audiences in school and higher education.
> (Marshall and Borrill, 1984, p.36)

They give an example of a youth worker who claimed that she had to contact young women before the age of 14 to have any hope of knowing them in the community-based setting as they grew older since, by 16, they 'disappear' unless some link has been made. The shadowy nature of their involvement is compounded by the resistance on the part of young men to sharing their space with young women and this is well documented in the study cited above.

Goggin (1993) notes that the concept of gay and lesbian adolescence is relatively new in relation to the study of adolescent sexuality and is related to the shift in assumptions about the nature of homosexuality being a pathological condition to less heterosexist perspectives. He concludes that:

> in these changing social contexts, however, lesbian and gay adolescents must surely be one of the most under-researched groups of adolescent and the most poorly understood in terms of sexuality.
>
> (Goggin, 1993, p.104)

Young women tend to be viewed as a problem in much research into youth but in distinctly different ways to young men. Media reports highlight how young women are perceived as endangering society by having children outside conventional family arrangements or by being considered as too young to be capable of instilling the appropriate values in their children. For example, Griffin, in a recent review of research on youth (1993), notes that in the USA interest in teenage pregnancy has in recent years tended to dominate the literature, replacing an earlier focus on teenage prostitution. This is supported by Moore and Rosenthal (1993) who also report that the paucity of information is at odds with current knowledge through crime reports about the increase in the numbers of young women prostituting in several countries. They also note that such statistics are likely to be inaccurate in terms of the actual numbers. Even less attention has been paid to adolescent male prostitution (McMullen, 1988).

Jesson (1993) reviewing literature on teenage prostitution, notes that very little has been written about issues of sexuality which concern young people in care. Similarly Whalen (1994) among others reports that young women who are survivors of sexual abuse are reluctant to use formal structures and official sources of help, turning instead to youth workers in a safe environment.

Young people who are using drugs may perceive this activity in completely different ways to professionals charged with educating them. Merchant and Macdonald (1994) undertook a small-scale study of Ecstasy users in the North of England, aged between 18 and 28, most of whom saw their use of the drug as purposeful and based on a balancing of the risks and benefits:

> Young people in the study argued that they were not ignorant in respect of the drug. They seemed reasonably well informed about its physical and psychological impact and took measures to combat some of the more frequent adverse affects ... They could talk about various health consequences of Ecstasy and other, newer drugs on the market. They knew the law surrounding Ecstasy and other drugs and the policing of raves did little to deter them from drug use. For young people like these, use of Ecstasy and other drugs has become a normal part of cultural life and they were happy and willing to discuss this with us.
>
> (Merchant and Macdonald, 1994, p.28)

This demonstrates some of the challenges facing those educating in community-based settings – within one area there may be a myriad of different levels of experience and maturity, patterns of behaviour and settings within which young people act and interact. Community-based interventions may have the potential to engage with these since schools provide limited opportunities to explore the views and experience of those adolescents who do not fit into the mainstream. Although much data may have been gathered *about* these groups, little information exists as to how *they* identify the issues facing them and the services available to them.

On the face of it, extending community development methods to work with youth provides a mechanism for both accessing and building on the experience of the diversity of youth cultures. Thus those who are traditionally excluded from mainstream health education may be more positive about an approach which is specifically targeted on their reference

129

group or peers. In this way young people with disabilities, the young homeless, those in care, young gays and lesbians, young people from minority ethnic groups, those whose parents or siblings use drugs and so on can take an active part in their own education. Rather than being marginalized, their experience can be legitimized and accepted as part of the range of experiences of young people.

It is evident that many of those young people already involved in, for example, drug-taking activity, perceive existing health education interventions based on prevention as largely irrelevant to them. The 'just say no' campaign is one which is frequently cited as being ineffective and marginalizing. Other examples abound of how young people rework messages which are seen as marginal and irrelevant and subvert educators' agendas to fit with their own perspectives. A selection of posters advertising the 'heroin screws you up campaign' (aiming to graphically demonstrate the horrors of heroin use) were highly prized by some young people as presenting an image they aspired to – pale and interesting as preferable to bronzed and healthy.

One approach which can be seen as attempting to counter the marginalization of some members of the community is that of 'harm reduction' approaches which have been tentatively extended from the field of alcohol education on to issues such as sexuality and drug misuse. Harm reduction is based on the assumption that some people will inevitably not be persuaded to give up a particular activity and that education should focus on rendering it safer by accepting this fact at the outset. The worker then has to build up a relationship of trust and mutual respect with those concerned and assist them to adopt practices which reduce the dangers to the person and her or himself and to others involved with her or him. This entails reconceptualizing the individual or group and accepting that they do act purposefully. The risk that users will continue to practise unsafe behaviours has to be accepted and a long-term strategy is implicit in this approach. Needle exchanges are one example of this kind of initiative. Clearly there are serious ethical and moral issues to be considered, but this perspective allows those taking part in the activity to contribute to the debate. A harm reduction approach takes on considerable political overtones when issues such as under-age sexuality and drug use are discussed (Ives, 1990a).

Fears exist that such messages may be wrongly targeted at those who have not indulged in illicit activity and that this may give out confusing messages. This may apply particularly to young people at different stages of maturity. In addition the political implications of being seen to condone illegal or socially unacceptable actions have resulted in professionals adopting cautious approaches despite awareness of the limitations of reliance on purely preventative strategies. It is a curiously paradoxical view of education that knowledge and understanding of different patterns and practice, sifting of evidence and exploration of approaches is viewed as potentially dangerous in relation to 'sensitive topics'. Nevertheless, it is clear that existing policies make the adoption of this approach problematic for educators who have to interpret a plethora of confusingly worded sets of guidelines while remaining within the law.

A community development starting point permits ownership of the issue, in that groups themselves negotiate a set of issues, and participate in each stage of the process. Providing safe settings for young people to explore further the range of issues facing them enables them to explore and analyse their different perspectives with a worker who has no formal authority over them. In this way the group experience can be taken account of and used positively to open up further discussion. Thus the possibility exists for the fostering of partnerships between professionals, policy-makers, parent groups and other young people. Health as a holistic process has therefore the potential to provide a means of examining and understanding complex sets of meaning and behaviour, within a non-judgemental setting.

Questions of territoriality may also be effectively addressed using community development principles and methods. Much detached and outreach work is based on the principles of community development, working mainly with disaffected young men on their own 'patch'. The use of staff who empathize and understand local language, contexts and cultural practices has been a long-standing (if under resourced) element of youth provision with its roots in the ethnographic research into delinquency pioneered by the Chicago school of sociology in the 1920s (Whyte, 1941). This school explored the sociology of youth in relation to 'the gang' which has remained a strong theme in youth research. Later analyses focused on social issues such as class and its impact on the lives and expectations of young people (Willis, 1977).

Detached work has traditionally been based on helping young people on their own terms within their own peer or friendship group. Although the group might be selected on the basis of their perceived threat to social order, the methods adopted in work emphasize the need to take a lead from their interests and issues and work with them on these. Health in its broadest sense may thus be one of many issues which will be addressed. A more explicit focus may prove attractive to younger groups but is heavily demanding in terms of workers' time and skill. Traditionally this work has focused on the most visible groups, mainly young men, with the interests of young women being seen as secondary and usually of lesser interest, as several critics have noted (Griffin, 1993; McRobbie, 1991). Young women's groups may also be more enthusiastic about participating in such an initiative which is focused on health, but where they have control over setting the agenda and defining the topics.

For professionals, work undertaken in this vein can also provide a means of gaining a more accurate insight and understanding of the contexts and realities of life for different groups. In this sense detached work may be a useful means of gathering information which fosters more effective collaboration between professionals and young people. By engaging with such groups and their needs health promoters and other educators can gain insight into the range of needs and go beyond working with those already motivated to adapt their lifestyle or who subscribe to health promoters' agendas.

A community development perspective can therefore address many of the issues facing health education at the present time. It may also serve to highlight serious deficiencies in provision and point to inequalities which structure young people's experience.

Problems with community development

It is clear that, despite the apparent potential of community development for working with young people, serious obstacles exist in implementing effective strategies based on this model. Some of these are practical considerations which have also bedevilled many health education initiatives. The underfunding and the marginal position of community development strategies in relation to departments and agencies is a key issue which has been noted by a number of commentators (AMA, 1993; Yates, 1994).

Linked to this, the reluctance of different professional groups to work collaboratively is a recurring theme. Although health may be theorized as a holistic concept this may be interpreted in widely differing ways by different professional groups, and even among practitioners within the same organization. There may be a multiplicity of vested interests held by different stakeholders which have to be forged into mutually acceptable strategies. These may demand compromise on several levels. Reaching agreement on the basis of clearly articulated 'mission statements' and approaches demands not only commitment and tact but also realistic understandings about expectations and ownership.

A clearly agreed and well-prepared initiative based on community development principles may in itself provide a vehicle for overcoming such obstacles at least at local levels. Such endeavours need to be reported and evaluated thoroughly on their own terms to enable future initiatives to avoid reinventing the wheel and to build on previous experience. The

133

question of evaluation of such work is also problematic. This method may provide insight for devising further strategies and has the potential to provide unique data on the contexts of young people's lives but for this to become the case then systematic recording, reflection and analysis is essential. Finding appropriate and user-friendly means of undertaking this may mean very different things to the different partners in the process. Moreover, appropriate forms of evaluation are also urgently required.

Other issues may be equally problematic. The very appeal of this method for young people itself underpins much of the uneasiness of some professionals. Peer educators, for example, have reported the difficulty some adults face in giving up power. The political dimensions of working with groups and establishing collective approaches may also be threatening. Moreover, encouraging critical perspectives to be incorporated into health education strategies runs against much of the current orthodoxy of health boards and educational bureaucracies. As Altman (1993) stresses:

> Good community education programs will almost inevitably contribute to the growth of political awareness, which is one reason why conservatives are so threatened by peer education programs. (Altman, 1993, p.10)

Working alongside, rather than on behalf of, groups may demand a radical rethink of professional attitudes and mores, not least, for instance, the retimetabling of work to provide services at times acceptable to groups and in neighbourhood contexts. This is only one of a range of dilemmas which face such community educators, who have been rather facetiously but aptly described as requiring the skills of a 'Renaissance generalist' (Dudley, 1993). The worker has to balance the various agendas and work *with* rather than *on behalf of* the group, while retaining a relationship with a managing body and possibly a line manager from a professional organization. In-depth knowledge of health matters may be less important than skill in working with groups and an ability to seek out such expertise, but this may be unacceptable to health professionals. Management strategies also need to take account of the messiness of the process, which is not easily absorbed into corporate structures. The political and ethical problems of this approach have been well documented in the reporting of the UK community development projects of the early 1970s (Green and Chapman, 1992). Overall this perspective demands clear policies and lines of accountability for the worker, and an employing agency which is prepared to accept critical comment on existing provision.

Many arguments about this method have focused on the dilemmas for practitioners – the dangers of creating paraprofessionals rather than developing critical appraisals of existing policy; the encouragement of dependencies on workers; the manipulation of agendas and groups to fit external agendas, and the dangers of going 'native' are all difficulties which fall into this category. The importance of appropriate training and support is therefore vital at all levels. It may be the case that indigenous workers are the most effective organizers within the community, able to secure respect and trust, being known as informal sources of advice and help, but their style and lack of professional qualifications may be an obstacle to their employment by statutory bodies. In many cases such workers remain on short-term contracts, paid on lower scales and unable to command resources within the agency.

A more intractable set of issues is concerned with the broad aims of this perspective – community development has been a feature of many community-based initiatives in the past twenty years but has often failed to 'deliver the goods' (Yates, 1994). The aims of such projects have often been unclear, the strategies muddled and the point of the exercise has often become lost in a mound of bureaucratic management structures which are poorly understood by all except inveterate 'meeting people'. It may also be a feature of its marginal position within agencies and the desire of some practitioners to maintain purity by remaining isolated from other professional

135

groups and focus on building links within communities. Another important but often neglected aspect is the poor and sporadic reporting of work by practitioners whose priority is, of necessity, grass roots work rather than theoretical analysis.

The question of appropriate time-scales and budgets is linked to the foregoing questions. This is possibly the greatest barrier to extending community development ideas into work with young people on a systematic basis. Attaching the term 'community' is often seen as a cheap option and a means of cutting costs. Community development, however, is highly labour intensive with its focus on small groups and the length of time required to build up community initiatives. There is also pressure to produce results quickly, a feature of the HIV/AIDS crisis which has demanded urgent and hasty answers to questions about behavioural change. Realistic time-scales need to be set for the development of community approaches with in-built evaluation.

Educationally, there are serious questions about how the method is described to young people – is it education by stealth and if so what are the implications? Alternatively should young people who are going through the processes of adolescence be burdened by having to take such responsibility for their own learning in their leisure time? It is clear that many young people are dissatisfied with what is on offer elsewhere but does this mean they really want to get involved in the tortuous process of community organizing? These questions will be tackled in more depth in the next chapter, but it is important to stress that there is evidence that this approach has a great deal to offer in channelling the energy, enthusiasm and abilities of many different groups of young people.

What is the place of health education in youth work?

Clearly the youth service in England and youth workers employed by community education departments in Scotland, interact with numerous groups of young people in informal settings. For many such workers, there is a strong educational

focus to their work and some of these adopt strategies which
are close to those identified in the previous sections as community development perspectives. The director of the National
Youth Agency gives the following definition:

> The youth service does, however, have a particular focus and value
> base. It starts primarily from a young person's perspective, and in
> the context of equal opportunity and participation is concerned
> with achieving individual or group change for the benefit of the
> young people concerned. (Paraskeva, 1991, p.231)

The Association of Metropolitan Authorities take a similar
view:

> The principles underpinning community development also under-
> pin youth work. Youth workers engage with young people where
> they congregate and work with groups of young people to tackle
> the issues which are affecting them. Most youth workers recognise
> their role as informal educators, very often working with young
> people who are alienated from school. (AMA, 1993, p.70)

In a similar vein, a recent HMI Report in Scotland defines
youth work as follows:

> Youth work comprises a wide range of educational activities which
> aim to provide young people with opportunities for personal and
> social development outside the formal system of education. It may
> take place in statutory or voluntary youth clubs, uniformed youth
> groups or even on street corners. Regardless of the setting its
> fundamental characteristic remains the same: purposeful interac-
> tion between adults and young people. When youth work is of high
> quality it has a clear educational content which is understood by all
> those involved. (HMSO, 1991, p.5)

Such a broad remit clearly leaves a place for health education
as part of the 'opportunities for personal and social development', but there is no specific case made for it. Health work is
often integrated into the day-to-day work of community
education organizations and it can be difficult to focus on the
'health elements' without imposing an artificial structure. In
actuality there is far from being a consensus on the ground

that health education *is* a legitimate part of the community worker's concern although this may be changing as informal settings become seen as legitimate sites for health education in the climate of HIV/AIDS (Hendry *et al.*, 1991). Some youth workers interviewed in a previous study retained an image of health education as being principally about 'hygiene and good habits' which they viewed as inimical to the kind of relationships they wanted to undertake with young people (Hendry *et al.*, 1991b).

Historically, there has always been a tension within youth work between its function in exerting social control over male working-class adolescents on the one hand and what is often lossely described as political education on the other hand. The provision of leisure facilities where youngsters can let off steam and take part in a range of activities is often in conflict with discussion-based work and exploration of values and beliefs. In the literature on youth a number of commentators have pointed to the tensions between leisure and education which are often experienced by young people themselves (Smith, 1988; Brake, 1980). This uneasy relationship between leisure and informal education continues to constrain attempts to tackle health education within youth work frameworks.

This vagueness about what constitutes legitimate youth or community work has often prompted suggestions of a more formalized curriculum underpinned by a sounder theoretical base. The arguments for and against generate much heat, if not a great deal of light. For those who oppose the more formal curriculum, its imposition is seen as inimical to the idea of being a service responsive to needs. However it may be more helpful to highlight the strands of youth work which offer the best promise of work on health-related topics rather than envisaging this as a feature of all interventions.

Smith (1988), in a review, suggests:

> In a sense it is more helpful to think of these being different and competing forms of youth work rather than a single youth work with common characteristics. (Smith, 1988, p.59)

The most recent study of the benefits of youth work (Hendry *et al.*, 1991) supports this view. In teasing out how health education is initiated and sustained within youth work it may be helpful to bear this in mind, especially since dominant models of youth work may not be the most appropriate mechanism for working with groups defined as being particularly at risk, or with a specific interest in certain aspects of health.

The position of 'alternative' youth work strategies other than the mainstream one is moot, however, and this is problematic for health education since it may be that it is 'alternative' youth work strategies that hold the best potential for effective interventions in relation to young people's health.

As Lightfoot and Marchant (1990) note in a recent review of youth participation in the community:

> There is relatively little written material on the subject of contacting young people who are not attracted to conventional youth activities. There is some written material on contacting the community in community work literature and while some of these approaches could be used with young people, others do not take account of their street life. There is also little in the literature that takes account of the cultural differences in making contact in the community. (Lightfoot and Marchant, 1990, p.14)

Evaluation of such different youth work initiatives is similarly uneven. A recent HMSO Report (1991) for example barely mentions detached youth work, small group work and work with girls. Where these are referred to, there is no indication of the aims and methods implied by such strategies. Nor is there any indication of how these activities are initiated, developed or evaluated in terms of their educational role.

Apart from that within specialized and especially feminist literature (McRobbie, 1991; Nava and McRobbie, 1984; Mountain, 1990) there is little written evidence that youth work encompasses much more than traditional youth clubs and to a lesser extent, detached youth work (Jeffs and Smith, 1990). Given that these initiatives may be the most fruitful, if small-scale, area for interventions on health education, serious gaps emerge in 'official' versions of youth work practice.

Much mainstream youth work continues to be based in large mixed settings, running in community centres, halls and churches (HMSO, 1991; Jeffs and Smith, 1990). The clientele is increasingly under 16, with older teenagers opting for commercial leisure provision (HMSO, 1991). Clubs are staffed by volunteers or part-time staff deployed by community education or voluntary organizations and supported by full-time professional workers. The terms of such support vary, as do the training opportunities and resources to run the clubs. The difficulties in recruiting and retaining part-time workers have been generally recognized as undermining one of the main aims of youth work, that of building trusting relationships between adults and young people.

The declining population of under-16s has been identified by the National Youth Bureau as having an important impact on the future development of youth work (Smith, 1990). The figures on which the report is based are English but the issues clearly also apply to the Scottish context. The report urges a rethinking of policies and provisions in the light of demographic change. The Scottish figures provided by Youth Clubs Scotland reflect a similar position although it is important to note that not all youth clubs or groups are affiliated to YCS (Shucksmith *et al.*, 1991).

Nevertheless the underlying assumptions of community development and youth work provide a useful starting point for creative forms of intervention with a wide range of young people. Rather than the 'quick fix' or 'hit and run' interventions which aim for immediate results, long-term strategic planning of interventions may also challenge the feelings of powerlessness experienced by some young people in relation to their health.

6 Reaching the young: alternative approaches

Introduction

The previous chapter has explored some aspects of community-based education with young people and some of the constraints on mainstream youth work in finding a place for health education. Nevertheless community perspectives can provide useful insights into reaching and working with groups and individuals who do not usually come within the orbit of health educators. For professionals and policy-makers these approaches can open up opportunities for feedback on pertinent issues and concerns neglected or overlooked by more conventional approaches. For young people, particular forms of youth work may hold promise for health education which recognizes differences and responds flexibly to their needs.

The first section of this chapter will therefore explore evidence of how some young people perceive their needs for health education. The next section will go on to consider first the particular example of peer education, drawing out dominant themes and examining the dilemmas posed by this approach for professionals and young people. The chapter goes on to explore detached or outreach work, youth advice and information services, and small group work with young people as examples of alternative ways of raising health issues with young people in community settings. Although in practice these approaches often overlap, it may be helpful to separate them in order to highlight particular themes and wider questions considered elsewhere in the book.

Young people's needs in health education

A recent study carried out by the authors (Hendry *et al.*, 1991) sought to meet with young people in a variety of community settings in order to explore their perceptions of health education and how relevant it was considered to be in relation to their needs and experiences. Thus in addition to working with young people within schools, a range of groups were contacted including: young homeless people recruited through a youth project, residents of hostels, members of youth groups, groups within intermediate treatment projects, young people living in care, young gay men and lesbians, college students and groups recruited through training agencies. The researchers did not attempt to identify these groups as 'representative' of the youth population but rather sought to investigate different levels of understanding and issues of importance to those interviewed. The aim was to gather textured and in-depth accounts of some of the health and social processes involved and to gain some understanding of mismatches which might occur between for example, young people's experience of drugs compared to that of the professionals charged with educating them.

Discussions with young people explored their levels of knowledge and levels of understanding about drugs and HIV. An important area of interest to the researchers was how young people felt about the health education that they had received.

Findings suggested that there was a consensus about the need for information that was accurate, up to date and 'relevant'. Often this was stated alongside criticisms of what had been offered to them by schools and parents. But the form they felt such education should take varied between and within the different groups. A number, mainly boys, felt they already knew enough about these topics but nevertheless many of these also felt much of the information that they received was confusing and ambiguous. Some believed that they learned most from experience and, while they were often critical of what friends might say, 'the street' was a ready resource, as one young man living in a hostel noted:

> You learn from the street. You read it. Pick it up. Everybody speaks about it, nearly every day.

In relation to drugs, some felt the information from schools was misleading and that it was actually confounded by their own experience and knowledge:

> They just give you warnings and you know there's more to it than that. Dope and acid aren't addictive – in fact dope is less dangerous than drink. If they told you more about what it does to you, give more details from nurses and folk like that ...

Parental knowledge was seen as inaccurate by some, but more often the relationship between parents and children made the home an inappropriate setting for education:

> I can speak to my parents – well my mother – about most things. But I wouldn't ask about some things, I'd definitely stick to safe areas.

For others there was a feeling that parents needed to be shielded from some of the realities of teenage life, reflecting a belief that parents' outdated knowledge made them likely to overreact out of fear of the unknown:

> My mum would mangelise me if she knew what I get up to. It's not that I'm that bad, she just doesn't have a clue about how things have changed.

Another commonly expressed feeling was that some parents have their own agendas when it comes to talking about sensitive topics. Because of this the information they give may be shrouded in mystery or ambiguity. For example many were seen as reluctant to recognize that young people are growing up and becoming active sexually:

> They don't want you to grow up like them – it's too late for them, but not for you.

Others felt that parents give 'mixed' messages which make their information suspect:

> Your father says, 'don't smoke' when he has a cigarette in his hand and, 'don't drink' when the following weekend he's out at the bar getting drunk.

Hypocrisy was often taken to be a feature of general adult attitudes towards young people and the phrase 'they've forgotten what they were like' was often repeated.

For many of those interviewed, health education, especially in relation to sexuality and drugs, drew parents into very artificial ways of trying to educate which were not applied elsewhere. Some young people were well aware when they were about to 'get the talk' and would prepare accordingly:

> Every time they go to a parents' night you can see it a mile off, they try to give me *A Talk* ... it's really funny.

When it came to discussing what parents and others should do, there was some consensus that 'outsiders' who have little connection with other aspects of their lives, have a clear educative role:

> Our education on sex was too late. I got chucked out ... for making dirty remarks, but nobody got the chance to speak and it was just boring ... they should get people who aren't teachers, who know what it is like and can take it.

There are several important points to be made which emerge from this quotation. Firstly it raises the question of what register is appropriate for discussion of sex. A number of studies (Ingham *et al.*, 1992) have shown that sexual terminology can be easily misunderstood, and terms used by teachers and others can be vague and ambiguous. Asking for clarification may leave the individual open to ridicule and abuse by others. Thus fears for their reputation might inhibit any acknowledgement of ignorance for many boys.

Secondly this participant also identified an 'outsider' as being more knowing and authoritative than teachers. It may also be that it feels safer to invest a 'stranger' with such status, since however knowledgeable and authoritative the teacher may be, she or he will have to be faced every day and have more power over the young person if they are acknowledged as 'expert' in this field. Young people are often well aware of the implications for teachers and others of disclosing sensitive information. A concern was also expressed that appearing too curious or aware could provoke unlooked for intrusions by teachers and loss of control.

Thirdly, the participant makes the plea for someone who is recognized as being in touch with the realities of teenage life, who can listen without embarrassment or judgement and who can sustain a climate of trust. This may seem a tall order but perhaps reflects the contradictory treatment accorded to young people as a group and to sexuality as a topic within this society at the present time. The theme of suitable adults who would be able and prepared to listen was raised on many occasions. This was not however as straightforward as it first appeared, since some young people had clear ideas about what they expected of such an adult and many contradictory qualities were cited. To some, for example, it was important for this person to be youthful and to have some 'street cred,' while others felt this was less important than the person having an ability not to impose their version of reality, while others felt some guidance was important. Essentially most argued for a person or persons who could empathize with young people without patronizing them.

The findings of this project have been echoed in a recent study undertaken by Fast Forward in schools and adolescent units in the Lothian Region of Scotland (Fast Forward, 1994). Here a team of young volunteers, aged between 18 and 25, supported by a trained worker distributed a questionnaire and organized group discussions on drug-taking and health issues over one year. The aim was to explore the information needs of young people in the 12 to 16 age group as a starting point for the development of appropriate strategies and materials. They discovered that despite some disadvantages relating mainly to

145

inexperience, the involvement of young people in the research study, was valid and was well received by participants. This innovative approach has raised many additional questions about the possibilities of peer research. They found that young people enjoyed learning about drugs and health through discussion but that certain criteria were seen as vital: being a stranger, not being an authority figure; having an open-minded approach; having potentially similar drug experience; having an awareness of street jargon; not being too much of an expert; being young. The research team points out that a combination of some of these factors was seen as preferable.

These themes relate closely to the desire expressed by many young people for some measure of control over the process of their own education. The wish for accessible and immediate help on the one hand and anonymous, confidential sources on the other are not as paradoxical as they might appear at first sight. Rather they reflect two dimensions of a spectrum of needs which may shift and move depending on a range of factors such as circumstances, nature of the issues, levels of support already used and relationships between young people and adults. Frequent comments about being able to speak about things and the need to feel safe and secure before approaching agencies demonstrate a serious gap in provision for young people. All this points to community-based initiatives as having the potential to work with rather than on behalf of the range of young people.

How well then, can community education address these learning needs in other realms of health education? We focus for the rest of this chapter first on peer education which is currently highly popular within health education. Despite its popularity, there has been little 'unpacking' of the advantages, disadvantages and dilemmas which it poses for educators and young people alike. After this we focus on a more general menu of youth work interventions which may represent a more sustained effort at understanding the realities of teenage life and addressing young people's health needs.

Peer education

Current interest in the concept of peer education in the UK has developed dramatically over the last four years. Developments in this country have drawn heavily on experience from North America and Australia where peer education is well established within a range of disciplines and settings (Wodak *et al.*, 1990; Kar *et al.*, 1986; Ovenden and Loxley, 1993). In both countries many peer education interventions have placed a strong emphasis on behavioural change, a point we will return to later.

The popularity of peer education in this country can be seen from the level of support now given to interventions by the Health Education Authority in England and its Scottish equivalent, the Health Education Board for Scotland. At both regional and local levels a host of short-term projects have also been established throughout the UK. Many of these are funded by the 'ring fenced' HIV/AIDS budgets of health promotion departments.

It is a strategy which has been identified as particularly likely to have success in working with those who have rejected more traditional approaches to health education but who are nevertheless defined as 'at risk'. This should be viewed within the context we have explored in earlier chapters where youth as a category is 'problematized'.

Despite the levels of this activity the term 'peer education' is poorly defined and existing interventions encompass a wide range of perspectives on young people, education and health (Milburn, 1994).

Peer education can be seen as a concept which acts as an umbrella to a wide range of terms – peer tutoring, peer teaching, peer coaching, peer learning, peer facilitating, peer educating, peer influencing, are just a few of those in use. Subtle differences exist between many of these relating to setting, perspective, aims, methodologies, target groups, recruitment patterns and time-scales. In some respects this diversity is exciting and demonstrates the level of interest and creativity sparked off by the idea. Conversely such diversity can also lead to confusion and uncertainty if there is no precision or agreement about the different meanings. Moreover, the adoption of the term by a disparate range of professional groupings and interests, all claiming it as their own and attaching their own sets of interpretations can result in further contradictions. There is thus a real danger that the term becomes so vague it loses meaning and usefulness. An urgent need exists to disentangle the dominant themes, establish some boundaries to the concept and examine it in depth to assess its value in working with young people.

Many peer education projects explicitly or implicitly share theoretical frameworks drawn from social psychology: in particular Bandura's work (1977) on role modelling and social learning has had an important influence. An acceptance that peer group norms are an important determinant of behaviour change is an important, if somewhat unproven, underlying theme (Swadi and Zeitlin, 1988). A further taken-for-granted assumption is that peers will be more acceptable purveyors of information since many young people claim to learn most from peers although they may express uncertainty about the quality of the information that is passed on. Within this scenario, peer education is clearly about discharging health education messages in ways which are more palatable to the client group. It may be that the messages will be modified by the peer educators to take account of context but the basic assumption is that they become agents for effective delivery of a specific set of messages in the hope of effecting behavioural change.

The health belief model of health (Ajzen and Fishbein, 1980; Fishbein and Middlestadt, 1990) with its emphasis on empowering individuals to take responsibility for their health and to build up and rehearse skills alongside peers has been influential. These theories are discussed more fully in Chapter 3.

But there are other bodies of research and theory which inform peer education in the broader context as the following examples illustrate. These are used to demonstrate that the notion of peer education may usefully move beyond a focus on individual change and assist in helping community change.

The idea of 'education for empowerment' has become a cliché in peer education circles. The work of Paulo Freire has influenced a number of interventions both in the USA and the UK (Wallerstein and Bernstein, 1988; Wallerstein and Sanchez-Merki, 1994; Kirkwood and Kirkwood, 1989). However few advocates of peer education have explored these links in depth. An exception is an intervention undertaken in Tayside in Scotland by Redman (1992) where an extensive consultation exercise with young people formed the basis for the establishment of Bodymatters, a group of young people who view peer education as a significant aspect of their work. Other aims of the group include establishing premises where health and information services for young people can be provided and extending membership of the group to others through newsletters and campaigning. Already successful in gaining funding for the centre, they describe the peer education element as:

> aiming to educate themselves about health and other issues, e.g. sex, contraception, relationships, age of consent, leaving home, abortion, adoption, alcohol – so that they can pass on correct information to other people. (Redman, 1994, p.9)

Feminist theory has also been influential in the development of initiatives such as the YWait project in Manchester, where young women with support from development workers have developed a drop-in health centre focusing on the needs of young women, providing medical services (including contraception prescribed by a doctor and nursing staff). The drop-in is a setting which young women can use informally to pick up information, discuss, find support or check out the agency. Peer education is a central element in the training of volunteers undertaken by established users. Thus peer education operates within this project at a range of levels: some takes the form of outreach work in schools, with youth groups and with professionals, but it also takes the form of volunteering to staff the

149

drop-in and making presentations at conferences. In this way peer education is a process in which the agenda is set to a large extent by the young women themselves.

In this project there is a blend of medical and non-medical services where health has become a focus of a partnership between young women and professionals. This project is funded and supported by health services, the local council and youth services, having recently secured core funding after three years of grant aid. Much work has been put into developing and sustaining a strong network of support within the area and with various agencies. It developed from work on 'well women' issues in North Manchester and was well supported by professional women working in health and youth work fields. It therefore has a strong element of self help and is thus a fairly equal partnership between medical expertise and the experience and identified needs of the young women themselves.

Both the projects cited above are atypical as far as health education sponsored peer education projects are concerned in that they incorporate some aspects of community development. Both have also had a relatively long period in which to develop their ideas and expertise. However they demonstrate the scope of peer education in community-based interventions.

A project which purports to offer a radical form of peer education is the more recently formed Crew 2000 based in Edinburgh. This peer coalition was formed by workers concerned about the lack of services offered to recreational drug users of the new 'rave' culture. They clearly identified this group of users as in need of help.

> In several ways the club dance scene is a risk-laden situation. Many of those involved are young, new to drug taking, and know little about the drugs they use.   (McDermott and McBride, 1993, p.13)

Provision of accessible information is the main focus and this takes a variety of forms including the distribution of condoms and leaflets. The underlying assumption is that the sub-culture of drug-taking has to be appealed to within the norms and values of the group. Based on an American model, the coalition is made up of workers and young people who attend clubs on a regular basis and who have a variety of skills, being students, artists, designers, DJs and unemployed. Leaflets have been designed and distributed, based on regional humour and with an explicit harm reduction message based on the comics produced by the Lifeline project in Manchester. They see their role as building up credibility within the club scene and argue, somewhat contentiously, that their approach can challenge the power differential between workers and drug users. A major principle of the coalition is to exclude anyone from the coalition who cannot control their drug use on the assumption that anyone who has such problems can offer little help to others. This project is in its early stages, having recently secured funding for shop front premises and it will be interesting to see how their model develops since it appears to be joining the ranks of the drugs agencies itself.

The projects outlined above have been selected to demonstrate particular aspects of peer education in the community. Interventions which follow a more conventional approach will be referred to in relation to specific questions and themes which are explored below.

Evaluation issues

A large number of peer educators have reported positively on the training undertaken, on the positive aspects of working as a group and being able to develop their own knowledge base (Fairmichael, 1992; Fast Forward, 1994; Dick, 1994). However there is, as yet, little reliable evidence of how this work impinges on the health attitudes and behaviours of the peer educators themselves, or of those who have experienced the peer education process as students. Findings from an action research study undertaken by the authors (Shucksmith *et al.*, 1995) tentatively suggest that using youth work methods and a community development approach within a neighbourhood context may offer the opportunity to engage

151

meaningfully with some of the issues facing groups of young people. However there is a need to be cautious about some of the claims made for this approach if it is to avoid being simply another short-lived fashionable concept.

Several critics have noted that the evaluation of peer education strategies in general remains uneven and problematic (Milburn, 1994). Supporters of the concept have tended to view peer education as a social movement and as such have displayed some reluctance to accept any criticism of the idea. Clear parallels exist in relation to the evaluation of community development, in particular the tension between becoming a recognized professional activity and a social movement (Thomas, 1983).

Moves towards the establishment of national organizations and the setting up of journals based on peer education demonstrate that peer education is assuming either *a* professional or *several* professional identities and these will provide vehicles for much needed debate.

To this end the large number of reports of peer projects will also be useful. The existence of these reports lies in contrast to the paucity of written up accounts of community-based interventions in general and may itself demonstrate the pressure to constantly justify the work and seek funding. It may also reflect the uneasy siting of projects within health authorities whose ethos and culture is more biased towards easily quantifiable forms of intervention. Whatever the reason these reports are often difficult to compare with one another and analysis of the relative strengths and weaknesses of projects remains highly problematic.

Peer education in youth work

A number of commentators have noted the similarity in aims between youth work and peer education (Clements and Buczkiewicz, 1993; Redman, 1988). The relationship may operate on different levels: a number of projects have been jointly initiated or developed alongside youth or community education services (as for example with Bodymatters in Dundee; East Cumbria Community Youth Project; Ayrshire and Arran Project). Many employ youth workers (Cambuslang Youth Health Project), and most draw heavily on youth work methods of working with young people (Clements and Buczkiewicz, 1993). In addition many, although not all, young people are recruited through their existing involvement in youth services and much of the work of peer educators takes place in youth work settings.

A principal difference between peer education and conventional youth work lies in the former's emphasis on a predetermined area of interest such as health rather than the open-ended negotiation of an agenda which characterizes much youth work. However it is often argued that if health is viewed as a holistic process, then scope for participants to negotiate the curriculum on health remains. For example in a recent study carried out by two of the authors (Shucksmith *et al.*, 1995) one (male) group decided to focus on drugs-related issues while another (female) selected sexuality and built up training programmes around the two topics. Participants in both groups had little time for health education on offer to them in school but were consistent in attending the training and showing interest in the issues. As groups they also identified clear differences between the generalist youth groups that they attended and the peer education training, commenting favourably on the 'learning' aspects of the project:

> It's a good laugh and you learn something. It gives a lot of information about stuff you don't know.

A local youth worker commented to the fieldworker about the boys' group:

> the attractions of risk, sex and drugs have now developed into an interest which they are developing using their own language and setting limits.

Within this project it rapidly became clear that any perceived

153

similarities with school styles of learning and operating would be unwelcome and that the processes of negotiation, control and participation were what stimulated enthusiasm in the project.

Another difference between peer education and more generic youth work is the multi-agency nature of funding for some projects which until recently was a small element of youth service funding. Where joint work has been successful, a great deal of preparation, planning and exploration of shared aims has underpinned the early work. In Ayrshire and Arran, for example, a multi-disciplinary group met for some time before the project itself began in order to identify shared principles and aims. In all too many peer projects, however, lack of understanding of the aims and agendas of the different agencies has resulted in tensions over the nature of the project. Often this has centred around an emphasis on measurable behavioural change by some stakeholders. Instances have been cited by fieldworkers of leaflets and posters produced by peer groups which then have to be ratified by this or that agency before agreement is made to give permission for use.

A further serious difference is the short time-scale many peer projects are working to, which nonetheless do not lead to lower expectations as regards output. As Clements and Buczkiewicz (1993) point out, peer education projects are seen as innovative and as such may qualify for 'pump priming' funding which may then not be available to continue beyond the first phase. Thus those working with the group and the group itself may be coerced into defending the project on spurious grounds simply to obtain further resource.

The attraction of peer education to health educators must be viewed in relation to the widely perceived failure of traditional modes of health education in dealing with so-called sensitive topics such as sexuality and drug misuse. In particular there is growing awareness that changes in knowledge do not necessarily lead to change in attitudes or behaviour and this has prompted the search for approaches which address these issues

(Gillies, 1989; Gatherer, 1979). As Fast Forward, one of the best known and respected peer projects states:

> Peer education is an approach which empowers young people to work with other young people and which draws on the strengths of positive peer pressure. By means of appropriate training and support, the young people become active players in the educational process rather than passive recipients of a set message.
>
> (Fast Forward, 1992, p.2)

Peer education offers the opportunity to tackle issues in a social context and takes account of holistic notions of health and illness. It also offers some promise in reaching populations which have traditionally rejected health education by working with, rather than in opposition to, existing peer groups, as with the Cambuslang project, which decided not to recruit selectively since:

> In many areas young people are not motivated to address health issues and would never have the confidence to stand up before their friends and impart information. Further, if we recruit those young people who are keen to do work then it may be that in this context, they are not credible sources of information. They have either taken on an adult role, replacing the worker as the expert or have become 'goodies'.   (Grant *et al.*, 1994, p.4)

Within the Cambuslang project the aim was to devise tasks with the young educators which would not disturb their credibility as the source of information but which would still guarantee the quality of information available. They would serve as educators only in their immediate surroundings, and would not be encouraged to see themselves as 'educators' in any para-professional sense.

The idea of peer education itself is of appeal in focusing on the positive aspects of youthful enthusiasm and enhancing this by intensive training which is then strengthened by a 'cascade approach' in work with other young people. It is envisaged that young people will then act as trainers to other young people either through presentations or informally in conversations.

155

Within the relatively young profession of health promotion the concept of peer education provides a mechanism for finding ways of capitalizing on local knowledge and tackling community as well as individual change. Such a move from the individual to the collective is a fundamental tenet of the New Public Health movement which was influential in developing the concept of health promotion as distinct from health education but which has remained elusive for health promotion departments. This movement based on the idealistic Ottawa Convention is oriented towards dealing with the structural constraints on health and tackling the sources of inequalities (Ashton and Seymour, 1988). It also has the potential to become 'socially transformatory' in the way described by Aggleton (1989).

As a way of educating it has offered an opportunity to move beyond traditional barriers in communication between adult and young person barriers by putting the adult in a facilitating rather than directing role with groups. The role of adults is negotiated within the project and may take different forms at various stages. This approach is well established within a range of teaching disciplines. However questions remain about how adult trainers discharge their role and how they see the limits to it.

In addition the peer education approach implicitly recognizes that non-professionals may have valuable insights and contributions to make in this field and highlights the importance of better understanding of lay belief, bringing young people into this arena and recognizing that they learn outside the classroom and bring their experience to understandings of health. It also gives the adults the chance to develop some insight into different forms of youth culture and in particular street life.

Who are 'the peers' in peer education?

The creation of élite corps of adolescent role models may further jeopardize the existing peer group relationships and further alienate disaffected young people. This raises the question of what exactly constitutes a peer? Is it someone of similar age, similar background, similar friendship group, or similar outlook? The answer to this remains vague in both the literature and in reports of peer education projects. Some peer projects do not work with existing peer groups at all. They may recruit from a peer group, selecting potential peer educators and training them within a close knit small group. Members of this group may develop peer affiliations to each other but this may well be mediated through the (adult) trainer. The peer groups with which they work may not be known to them at all before they are 'booked' for a session or series of sessions and in any case their first line of accountability may be to this new trainer.

Within specific, clearly identified communities of young people such as those who have 'come out' as gay, peer education takes on a different form, providing a means of validating experiences, sharing information and support and reinforcing a sense of community. With some groups of drug users there may be similarities as a consequence of all being involved in an illicit activity: Coffield and Gofton (1994) point to evidence which suggests that, in contrast to dominant stereotypes, many young drug users are the pace setters, the favourites, the peer leaders who wield considerable influence and who may be able to work effectively within peer groups. Should peer education, then, focus more clearly on particular groups which may be aware of the risks, knowledgeable about health but find putting this into practice poses unacceptable risks in other areas of their lives? Young women's groups may also have shared experiences and sets of values which dispose them favourably to this approach and may give them insight into the difficulties which other groups of young people face, but will this be true of *all* groups of young women? Should peer education focus rather on those barriers or difficult groups, and work, for instance, with groups of young men to challenge 'macho' attitudes and behaviour which serve to marginalize those who do not accept this model or who are put 'at risk' by it?

157

The process of selection of peer educators itself inevitably alters the structure and relationships within a peer group. It is clear from a number of reports of projects that some trained peer educators are reluctant to undertake an explicitly educational role within their own neighbourhood or area. (Grant, *et al.*, 1994). And yet it is assumed that a principal aim of this form of intervention is to respond to locally defined needs and issues which are assumed to be more accessible to peer educators than professionals.

Although it may be a process which has potential for working with the disaffected or alienated populations of young people, it is clear that many peer projects also principally attract the articulate and confident who are relatively successful within other contexts. Fast Forward for example recruits from a wide geographical area and adopts a roadshow approach which often builds on local groundwork and provides a stimulus for the future by alerting agencies and young people to health issues and the potential of a peer approach. Peer education projects in school settings tend to recruit from the upper echelons of the school, on the basis that these students will provide acceptable role models.

> Many acclaimed examples of this practice have a high level of motivation amongst the young people. The young people are often middle class, academic achievers who are confident and open to the training techniques that are employed.   (Grant *et al.*, 1994, p.1)

Working with more disaffected young people clearly presents a powerful set of challenges for peer educators, yet it is here where the most significant inroads are possible in addressing the context and dilemmas posed to young people.

There is a possibility, however, that such an approach, handled insensitively, may 'set young people up to fail', as the workers in the Cambuslang project indicate when they suggest that peer educators used in 'traditional' ways would be seen as taking on an adult role, replacing the worker as 'expert' or become 'goodies'.

Often young people are reluctant to work with their own

peers as was found in the Aberdeen study where the young men especially felt this would be unacceptable. This was for territorial reasons while with other projects it was more lack of confidence.

> The play was successfully completed but the girls were too embarrassed to perform to their own peers.　　(Grant, *et al.*, 1994, p.2)

It may also be a feature of being seen to take on a role which is not in keeping with the identity already formed by the young person with their immediate peers.

Selecting and training 'peers'

There are at least two distinct stages which need to be accommodated by both the group and the trainer – the training stage where young people are recruited and educated to some degree over several weeks or months. In many accounts it is clear that this is a fairly intensive process where strong relationships are built up. The second stage entails the provision of support and backup to the group as it sets about training other groups. It could be argued that these demand quite different kinds of qualities and skills if the group is to make a smooth transition. Within some groups there will be processes of selection and rejection which further complicate the process and pose dilemmas for the adults involved.

The enthusiasm and commitment of those who take part in peer education training is well known and possibly one of the most commonly accepted successes of such interventions (Goodlad and Hirst, 1989; Dick, 1994; Fast Forward, 1992 and 1994). There may be a number of reasons for such enthusiasm.

Firstly peer education projects may give an opportunity for young people to meet and discuss 'real issues' in their lives with non-judgemental adults in a setting where they are assumed to have some useful contribution to make. The novelty of this must be a reflection on how restricted interaction between adults and young people is outside formal or family settings:

What we really need in order to improve our learning is contact with adults other than parents and teachers; we know what our parents think, we know what teachers think and they're paid to do that. But what do real adults think?   (Abbott, 1994, p.93)

Peer education also holds out the possibility that young people can have some control over the agenda and style of the intervention. In a project undertaken by the authors, all the participants commented favourably on this aspect of the process which allowed their interests to determine the scope and pace of the training (Shucksmith *et al.*, in press).

It may further provide a chance both to use 'illicit' knowledge and to challenge orthodoxies as with the Crew 2000 project based in Edinburgh. This group uses a harm reduction approach to recreational drug users. The Edinburgh Stonewall group, set up to meet the needs of young gay and lesbians in Edinburgh, similarly has a remit to challenge dominant homophobic attitudes and support young people in coming to terms with their sexuality.

Most project reports cite the growth in self-esteem among peer trainers as a measurable outcome of the approach. Many projects point to reports of participants confirming this (Dick, 1994; Guy, 1991; Long, 1991; Fairmichael, 1992; Fast Forward, 1994). However it remains unclear whether it is the peer training process in itself which fosters this or aspects of the process such as being recognized as having something positive to offer or having control over some element of the learning process in a social context where some other young people feel disempowered. It may also be the case that young people gain a high level of social support from working as part of a team. It is equally unknown whether this growth in self-esteem and confidence is sustained after the intervention.

Involvement in the training programme itself is usually an affirming experience, confirming to the young person that they have strengths which may have gone unrecognized in other areas of their lives. Being involved in a small group and being recognized as offering a useful contribution may also boost confidence.

For many this overlaps into forming an acceptable identity and persona; this may be especially important for those previously judged lacking in formal educational settings, but who feel they nevertheless can communicate and do have something important to say. However, as yet there is little knowledge about those young people who drop out of peer projects or who feel such involvement is not for them. For example, Dick (1994), in her evaluation of the work of the Brook Peer Education Report, refers to the fact that after several meetings with potential peer educators, only two of the original group remained, but gives no explanation of this, merely indicating that others were recruited to the project. Elsewhere in the report, she indicates that the group tends to be self-selecting, and again it would be helpful to find out how this process operates. Data on how those who are not selected to undertake peer education perceive themselves and their abilities would also provide useful insights into the processes of peer education. In the authors' study one young woman decided not to take part since she felt she already had enough knowledge and provided peer education informally anyway (Shucksmith *et al.*, in press).

Increase in knowledge and understanding of health issues among the volunteers is clearly an important outcome, but one which is notoriously difficult to assess. However if young people are alerted to health issues through a project and, just as importantly, identify health as having relevance to their present lives, this may provide openings to develop an interest in other areas of their lives. In reality there is a vast difference between the ways in which training courses are undertaken, their content and styles of working. Some may offer the opportunity to explore personal issues and problems with relationships, while others will tend to focus on the provision of accurate information and advice on specific topics.

The role of the adult worker is a vital component of the process and the skills required of them often to go beyond training to include the administration, transport, securing of resources and dealing with managing bodies for the project and lobbying within agencies for support (Hamilton, 1992). In addition trainers have to strike a balance between empathizing and supporting on the one hand and on the other acknowledging and dealing with dependency where it exists so that the group retains its autonomy.

Ideally the experience will validate and reinforce the attitudes and beliefs of the peer group but there is the likelihood that the messages being given by trainers are rejected in favour of maintaining existing forms of credibility and behaviour. Groups may have their own agendas which they will argue for and pursue and which may be at odds with those of the trainer or the sponsoring agency.

Involvement in a peer education project may enhance young people's credibility and standing with peers but this again is double edged: in some cases it may have the opposite effect, drawing young people away from the original peer group and making it impossible to return. For some young people the implications for other aspects of their lives may be unacceptable. In the study conducted by Guy in Newcastle (1991) one young peer educator expressed heartfelt resentment at being approached in his 'time off' in the pub by young people who had been trained at a training session and wanted to talk about the issues when the trainer just 'wanted to get pissed'.

Supporting peer education initiatives

The perceptions and understandings of those who have been 'peer educated' also remain poorly understood. Many peer projects fail to move forward from the training element and a variety of reasons lie behind this. Many, as has been noted above, are funded on a short-term basis and in many cases the training element takes longer than anticipated. This is particularly the case in neighbourhood projects where a range of factors may intrude on the process. In the study undertaken by the current authors, for example, (Shucksmith *et al.*, 1995) the boys at a later stage claimed to be frightened to use the community centre which had become the territory of an opposing group. This situation was remedied by meeting in the house of one of the boys, though this took some time to organize. However it proved the point that the group wanted to continue their training and that the workers were prepared to negotiate with them. It also demonstrated the need to recognize the 'territory' of the group, not only in terms of sharing control over the process of training but also in relation to potential peer education training at the next stage. Similarly the training aspect sometimes had to be put to one side to explore some personal problems a member had to work through with the group. In this way the private problems became public and part of the process as inevitably they were concerned mostly with relationships, health concerns and worries. While both these examples hinge on what might be seen as peripheral issues, they demonstrate how initiatives within a community can be dogged by factors which determine how the intervention develops. In the authors' project these became part of the material of the project, strengthening relationships both within the group and between the group and the workers, as well as demonstrating a recognition of the context within which the young people lived.

There are other ways in which the second stage may be problematic. A number of examples demonstrate how the peer educators become reluctant to try their skill out within their local community and among their own peers. This raises some fundamental questions about which are the legitimate audiences for peer educators. In some cases it appears to be professionals themselves rather than young people who are most impressed by and responsive to the way peer educators work. Certainly many inputs to conferences by youth groups have been well received.

There are clearly strong contradictions in the peer education approach: peer educators, for example, may have undergone intensive training within a small group, over a period of months where their own views and values provide a good starting point but they may then go along to a youth club to deliver a one-off session where building such a rapport must be accomplished within an hour or so. In such settings it is difficult to get away from simply providing information rather than exploring issues in young people's own language.

Peer education: its future?

It is clear from this short review that there are questions posed both by the idea of peer education itself and by how it is practised. If it is to fulfil its promise of providing an effective as well as a flexible and enjoyable approach to health education with young people, these questions demand serious consideration.

Firstly there is the question of who sets the agenda and how different agendas are reconciled. For many educators it is clear that peer education is first and foremost a means of refining the bluntness of health education messages, providing an alternative means of manipulating peer pressure. Within this model there may be conflicts about target groups, about styles of delivery and about the level of sophisticated education offered as opposed to simply information-giving which is to be carried out.

Are peer educators able to go beyond the provision of information, albeit information which is more street oriented, more user-friendly and accessible? The sophistication of the training process and the intensity which is generated by, for example, discussion of issues and dilemmas around sexuality may be inappropriate in a youth club setting even if peer educators have developed the skills.

In general however, the principal model of peer education seems to reinforce notions that the mass of young people lack information, are socially incompetent and are thus simply in need of an injection of culturally specific messages. The emphasis on the learning of social skills to resist peer pressure suggests that the individual is open to be contaminated or cured by peers, rather than being a purposeful actor able to reflect and act.

Is there then a problem that peer education projects could simply be a repackaging of old messages in a new format? If this is the case it is a duplicitous strategy simply inviting young people to reproduce in a more acceptable form the failed messages of existing mainstream health educationalists.

Peer education may be a valuable asset within a wider programme – it can capitalize on the street contacts, street knowledge and the very real abilities of young people. Skilful work may be needed to ensure that this is a realistic goal.

However it demands a particular set of circumstances, skills and managerial support. It may require long-term funding and support. It may demand an ability on the part of administrators and funders to take criticism, to reconceptualize young people as potentially having valuable insights and experience rather than as essentially problematic. Neither should it be assumed that all young people will be receptive to this form of education. Young women may be able to talk to their peers about sex as Moore and Rosenthal (1993) suggest but this does not mean that peers will provide education on these topics. It may be one source among many and may be a way of rehearsing problems already raised elsewhere.

Peer education may offer an innovative way of working with young people and it has great potential for exploring many aspects of how young people learn. However there is a clear need to unpack and examine underlying assumptions and evaluate interventions. The claims made for the concept demand careful investigation if it is to offer a meaningful form of intervention.

Youth work interventions

Within the broad term of youth work lie a diverse range of interventions and there is no intention here to catalogue these since they are well documented elsewhere (Smith, 1988). In this section some dominant themes will be explored and illustrated using examples of initiatives which either have a particular health focus or have the potential to be adapted for work on health issues. Youth work is undertaken by a diverse range of groups and individuals but here we will focus mainly on interventions designed and undertaken by youth workers employed by local authorities or voluntary organizations which have an explicitly educational emphasis.

Much mainstream youth work continues to be based in large mixed settings, running in community centres, halls and churches (HMSO, 1991; Jeffs and Smith, 1990). The clientele is increasingly under 16, with older teenagers opting for commercial leisure provision (HMSO, 1991). Clubs are often staffed by volunteers or part-time staff deployed by statutory or voluntary organizations and are supported by full-time workers. Although great stress is laid on the educational role of youth work, the difficulties in recruiting, training and retaining part-time staff have been recognized as undermining this process.

The declining population of under-16s has been identified by the National Youth Bureau as having an important impact on the future development of youth work (Smith, 1990). However this decrease in numbers may offer opportunities for more developmental strategies to be adopted and for those approaches which have been at the periphery to assume greater prominence. It is such alternatives to the large youth club which may also offer most promise for health education initiatives.

Detached and outreach work

In the UK detached youth work was developed in the 1960s in the wake of the Albermarle Report (HMSO, 1959) as an innovative attempt to reach the 'unclubbables' or the 'unattached' who were reluctant to participate in conventional youth service provision and who were often regarded as posing a threat to the stability of society either by their riotous behaviour or rejection of conventional lifestyles (Morse, 1964; Smith, 1988). It was an early attempt to work with young people on their terms rather than setting out a stall of what was perceived as 'good for them'. Within a context where the idea of 'youth culture' was assuming great importance and media attention, detached youth work represented a way of reaching out to young people, in particular young men. Thus it is based on a deficit model of young people, and attempts to build on their own experience and complement this with input from youth workers.

It will be useful to make some distinction between detached and outreach work since these terms are not always interchangeable. Detached work often applies to working on the streets or 'where young people meet' with those who have no desire to use the services of community or youth centres. They may also work with those who are not welcome, for one reason or another, to use existing provision. On the other hand, 'outreach' is more often a term which describes work aiming to encourage better use of existing premises and services. Outreach workers work with groups who wish to use services but feel excluded by other users, staff or the ethos of the facility on offer. They may also work with those who are unaware of the service on offer. Thus there may be some overlap between the groups worked with by detached and outreach workers.

Many community-based interventions aim to work *with* peer groups and often build up contact with either one friendship group or a network of groups within a given area or neighbourhood. The youth worker makes contact with an individual or group on their own territory and with a minimum of 'props'. Initial work focuses on building up relationships and trust with the group. Thus the youth workers operating in this setting are likely to be grilled about their presence on the street, their plans, and importantly, their relationships with other agencies like the police and social workers who may be viewed with suspicion and hostility. Barrigan (1993) outlines this process in an account of health work carried out by staff from a detached youth work project in Newcastle:

> Workers find themselves making contact with young people on street corners, around pubs, fish shops and amusement arcades. Relationships are established through the service offered and

167

advice, support and direction can be enhanced. When trust and confidence has grown myths can be explored and attitudes challenged. Social and outdoor education can be programmed into the work for individuals and groups alike. The idea of the [health] project came directly from using this approach.

(Barrigan, 1993, p.67)

Acceptable reassurances about their trustworthiness may only be accepted as the presence and roles of the youth workers on the street becomes more established and distinct from that of other adults who are likely to be interested in the group. She or he may be tested out in different ways by group members and be placed in situations which demand a high level of skill, tact and judgement. They may be able to help with information on a range of topics but it is how this is handled that will determine how the relationship is framed and built on. The educational element of the work is constantly under negotiation between worker and group as one element in a complex mixture of issues and concerns.

The aim is to work primarily with the group on a collective basis rather than exclusively with individuals, although inevitably there is an interplay between these. Nevertheless, the focus is taken off the individual to some extent by recognizing the group itself as having responsibility and power to make decisions and carry them out. The worker may simply act as a foil for the group, listening and 'hanging about' with them, perhaps providing transport or some administrative help. The agenda of the worker is to help the group identify an aim, interest or issue, and work with them to achieve it, whether this be the organization of a trip, a discussion about drug use or negotiation of the use of premises to meet. A key element of this process will be negotiation over the respective roles of group members and youth worker. In this respect there is a clear distinction between the peer group trainer and the youth worker in that the latter has to some extent to develop a curriculum with the group while the former already has a curriculum planned and negotiation is over how this will be delivered.

168

Problems with the approach can arise should a group simply reject the overtures of the worker. In this case they simply will not appear at the usual times and places. More likely there may be some disagreement within the group as to the acceptability of having the worker around. Both workers and young people may develop a way of recognizing appropriate times to be around and may develop patterns of exclusion and inclusion. In this way skilled workers may manage their involvement and potential conflict with the group. Often the worker will be drawn into helping with various welfare rights, housing, employment or relationship issues. It is in this way that work around health issues may be tackled, but it is unlikely this will happen until some climate of trust and a belief that this is a suitable place to raise such issues is shared by worker and group.

A range of problems face detached workers in the building, sustaining and closing of relationships with individuals and groups but in some situations problems arise because of inadequate resourcing of the initiative and the lack of a long-term perspective. Adequate management structures and support networks are often absent leaving the workers isolated from mainstream youth work and liable to 'burn out'. Such an approach is difficult to accommodate within corporate management structures which may explain why interventions are often short term and developmental in nature. The lack of a base and the maverick nature of detached work demand skilled and flexible management which may be problematic within cumbersome local authority bureaucracies. The lack of understanding of this approach within management can also lead to poor framing of initiatives so that youth workers may be 'set up' with overly ambitious aims. Changing patterns of youth activity may also demand creative approaches to detached work, as for instance in meeting the needs of young women with children. Mountain (1985) vividly describes some of the difficulties in recruiting and working with such a group and goes on to explore some of the ways in which confidence, self-esteem and skills were developed.

169

Detached workers may also face difficulties in developing relationships with other workers; conflict is most frequently reported with police who may see the worker as colluding with illicit activities of groups (Lye, 1988). Similarly, young people may be suspicious of co-operation between detached workers and professionals such as social workers or health visitors. Some of these issues can be resolved through clear guidelines and management structures which may require a considerable degree of tact and sensitivity.

In recent years there has been a great deal of interest in developing outreach work in relation to prevention of HIV. This method has been used by a number of drugs agencies in attempts to reach hidden populations. Work tends to fall into two distinct patterns – that of bringing services to hidden populations of users on the street or outlying housing estates or as a mechanism for encouraging wider use of existing services (Rhodes *et al.*, 1991; Rhodes, 1994). Rhodes (1994) suggests that while outreach may make possible contact with some people who are in need, it remains a limited strategy for tackling more seriously 'hidden' populations. Within youth work the two strands are clearly visible: some youth centres have turned to street work as a means of increasing the numbers of clients of services while others have seen it as a means of addressing populations who have rejected centre-based services.

Youth advisory services

In recent years there has also been an increasing number of shops and centres providing information and advice to young people, and these appear to offer a valuable resource in terms of providing information about services etc. Some such as Off the Record, a well-established shop front in Stirling, Scotland, aim:

> to empower young people and to promote their personal and social development through the provision of an innovative information, advice and counselling service.   (Off the Record, 1992)

The drawback to this approach is the difficulty in building on the contacts made in the absence of group work. It is clearly the case that adult-based information services do not serve youth well and some issues in particular are neglected. The continued demand and support for Brook Advisory Services demonstrate this very clearly in relation to sexual health and contraception.

A basic decision facing a youth advisory service at its outset is whether or not it must aim itself at all young people or at particular target groups. Services established by statutory agencies may be under pressure to be all things to all people. There is insufficient resource to establish a service dedicated to a small sub-section of the population; therefore the agency must have broad appeal. The identification of a specific service for youth is a concession already in terms of slicing the potential catchment for a service within an area and dedicating resource to it.

In reviewing the provision of youth advisory services in both England and Scotland it is clear that their designation or the targeting of their remit must perforce pay attention to what services exist already. A case must be made for funding a new agency on the grounds that the existing ones do not address the needs of a significant group within the marketplace for advice. In some cases, as in the case of Off the Record in Stirling, the claim is that young people in general are not well served by existing general advisory services in the city. In others, as in the case of the Brook Advisory Centres, the justification for their existence lies in the neglect by other agencies of advice and particularly services on sexual health and pregnancy. Base 51 in Nottingham bases its claims for recognition and funding not on the grounds that other agencies do not exist locally catering for young people or covering health issues but on the notion that these are not attractive to a significant portion of the population who must be reached. Moreover, Base 51 is unique in spelling out its philosophy of a holistic approach to health in its work with young people (Shucksmith *et al.*, 1993).

171

Identifying the level and pattern of existing services and clarifying the market niche that such an agency will fill is an important step in the establishment of a service. Many agencies will incorporate their conclusions in the form of aims and objectives, and will gear their operation specifically to such target groups. Gender, social disadvantage, race, sexual orientation or ethnicity may all be the basis of targeting within the youth population, as might physical or mental disability, or the pursuit of particular 'risk' behaviours (e.g. drug or solvent misuse).

Age targeting is a real problem for such agencies. 'Youth' covers all ages from 12 to 25, yet the health needs (particularly in relation to sexual health) across this age span may be very different. Legal difficulties, fear of parental disapproval, as well as a disinclination to receive a negative press, may deter some agencies from marketing themselves towards under-16s. Other groups have secretly welcomed an apparently negative newspaper 'blast' for supplying under-age young people with contraceptive advice, precisely because it advertises the openness of their service to other young people in a way that they would find difficult to accomplish overtly. This has been the experience both with the Brook Advisory Centre in Belfast and with the Teenage Clinic in Nottingham in the past.

Some agencies will target according to the range of issues on which they will offer advice or assistance. In many cases workers interviewed on the range of services they offered noted how difficult it was to set boundaries around the issues with which they dealt. A young person with an initial enquiry about a housing problem might turn out to have a problem with a relationship that was ultimately of a sexual nature. Workers need to have the flexibility to operate across such a range of issues as well as to know when expert advice is needed and to whom they might make referral. Because of this many youth advisory agencies prefer to have a 'generalist' image, believing that young people have difficulty both in diagnosing the root of their own problems in many cases, and of presenting intimate or difficult problems to professional workers. Young people will test out the agency with a trivial problem before entrusting them with a major one. Such an approach characterizes the operation of agencies like Off the Record and Nottingham's Base 51.

The danger in such a generalist approach is that the agency may not inspire the confidence in young people to raise issues that aren't obviously highlighted. A service which does not specifically put health to the forefront of its remit, for example, may be seen as insufficiently expert or confidential to be consulted on such matters.

The obverse, of course, is that an agency too closely identified only with health issues runs the risk of missing those young people whose problem is essentially social in nature despite having implications for health. A young girl being pressurized into sexual intercourse before she is ready is not likely to identify her need as a health one, for example. To this we must add too the danger of an agency solely identified with health developing a white-coat, specialist image which will not appeal to the majority of young folk.

So far in this section the phrase 'targeting' has been used to signify the process where an attempt is made to clearly define the catchment for the service and to gear the agency towards the fulfilment of the needs of a particular segment of the population.

In some cases that were reviewed within this study, however, the target group was identified as *all* young people and this objective was pursued with a vigour which gives a whole new meaning to the concept of targeting. In Liverpool, for example, the Healthline project highlights different geographical segments of the city in sequence and goes into the area on a 'blitzkrieg' approach over a period. In Lothian Region, the *Schools' Sessional Workers' Project*, having been content initially to respond to school requests for their services finally took the bull by the horns and targeted instead those schools which did *not* use them, wanting to know why, and then tailoring the approach to suit. Now the community education service in Lothian is in the process of appointing a community education officer to work alongside the schools team so that particular geographical areas can be targeted.

These issues about targeting raise immediately the question of how an agency is to present itself to young people. The last two examples offered demonstrate a very proactive role, but most agencies operate on a much more responsive or reactive model, waiting for customers to come to them, or on a mixed model where a basically reactive format is spiced with a measure of outreach work.

Many agencies surveyed in the course of this project noted the importance, if they were going to sit back and wait for young people to nominate themselves, of offering an attractive and 'upbeat' image. They did not want to be seen as places where 'only young people with problems' went. To get a reputation as a place which catered mainly for 'junkies' or those down on their luck was to risk rejection by the majority. Such a paradoxical position is hard to maintain, making sure that those at greatest risk are catered for without alienating the bulk of the youth population.

The public image of an agency is nurtured, not least in part, through a name (Off the Record, YWait, Shades, Pulse, Jigsaw) designed to appeal to young people, through the design of its premises and through its advertising. Part of the reason why naming is so important relates to the role that such an agency often plays as a mediator between the individual young person and the 'unacceptable' face of a statutory authority. Even where regional authorities or health boards are the chief funders of a project, there is a felt need to give the agency its own clear identity and to dissociate it from other services or from the hint of official authority. Many vulnerable or 'at risk' young people already have cause to fear agencies like the Department of Health and Social Security or even the social work department. A simple example would be the young woman with a child who fears she may have HIV but is reluctant to seek help or testing for fear that the information will be divulged to the social work department and her children taken into care.

Premises for such agencies range from stark offices in dreary Victorian buildings, through renovated churches (Off the Record in its early days) to upbeat shop premises (Off the Record in its current manifestation) and, at the most expensive end of the market, to the purpose-built (or at least, purposefully converted) premises of Base 51. It is impossible to evaluate the appeal or relative effectiveness of such formats. What repels one group by its tackiness may appeal to another by its informality. What looks smart and upbeat to one crowd may look clinical, over-smart and forbidding to another. What is clear is that agencies can suffer guilt by association. Settings in existing health centres set a tone which no amount of renaming or overt denial can efface. Even if an agency cannot appeal to all groups, it perhaps ought to be afforded the opportunity to stand alone and make its own reputation.

Those agencies which have sought to create a reputation by advertising have quickly (or slowly) discovered that the best way of spreading their reputation is by the informal networks and word of mouth contacts among young people themselves. Agencies contacted in the course of the study described in Shucksmith *et al.* (1993) had used posters, cinema and newspaper adverts, handbills, stunt promotions, open days and so on. While such means may bring the existence of an agency to young people's notice, the decision to use the service, as young people confirmed in interviews, is often made in consultation with a friend and will be based on shared knowledge of their likely reception. Word of mouth reputations, however, take some while to establish. One of the problems of such agencies discussed later is the uncertainty of their funding from year to year and their reliance on evaluations of the service to secure more money – evaluations which take too little account of the time taken to build up a reputation among local youngsters for being helpful, non-discriminatory, expert and confidential.

Image, however, is also conveyed to young people through methods of operating. A traditional treatment-based model, for instance, might use a system of designated clinics and appointment times made in advance as a pragmatic response

175

to the need to maximize the use of the expensive services of medical personnel. The message is not wasted on the young person that a meeting so arranged is one where expert meets patient, where time may be limited, however serious the problem, where the problem will be defined and an attempt made to prescribe a remedy, where the fault or the problem lies with the presenting patient, and so on.

An agency determined to play down this 'medical' model might aim to operate on a 'drop-in' basis (with appointments only needed for people being referred on to others), and to offer a non-specialist 'ear' and an opportunity not limited by time to talk through general issues rather than specifically personal problems.

Some agencies find themselves driven from the second of these models back into the first by funding too limited to allow extensive opening times, by security fears about the danger to workers presented by clients (in the case of some agencies ministering to drug users), or by passing drunks and crackpots (many agencies are situated in urban locations which make them vulnerable during evening opening particularly). Financial constraints or fears for workers' safety are real and cannot be ignored, but so too is the impact on a young person with a problem of having to find a way to a back street location, having to locate a first-floor office by a small plaque outside in an alleyway and then to have to negotiate access to the receptionist via an entry phone.

Those agencies which operate proper outreach programmes offer an extension of the static image of the project base and can give alternative routes for access into the service, but most agencies see the need to adopt small-scale or short-term outreach in order to draw young people in. Off the Record, for instance, is essentially a drop-in or responsive service, but at different times volunteers have been involved in a number of initiatives, carrying out questionnaire surveys, leafletting in fancy dress and so on, to draw the project to young people's attention. Outreach sessions offered in schools also have real impact in conveying to young people the flavour of the welcome they might receive at the agency.

Other agencies have organized special events or theme weeks with exhibitions and presentations to draw young people in. Once over the threshold or in contact with agency personnel, even in a trivial encounter, the easier it will be the next time for the young person to make contact when faced with a real problem.

Small group work – single sex groups

The development of work with girls in the 1970s has had a strong and lasting impact on youth work as a whole. Women workers, often part-time, identified a need to challenge the existing domination of facilities and resources by males and to address the needs of young women more effectively. This demanded a critical evaluation of how gender influences and structures the experience of young women. The setting up of groups was itself problematic, involving many debates and arguments as the groups were often interpreted as 'divisive' by both full-time and part-time male staff as well as boys themselves (Spence, 1990).

Interventions take a variety of forms: 'safe spaces' within existing youth club sessions, the taking over of youth centres for an evening for young women and girls' days were also developed. Tension existed between the organizing of activities which were seen as reinforcing traditional 'women's matters' – the hairdressing and make-up syndrome – and more adventurous activites. Girls' nights however have offered opportunities to explore a range of issues and concerns with women workers in a supportive setting which was a means of confronting gender stereotypes. Inevitably issues around relationships, sexuality, health and well-being have been at the core of this form of intervention. The development of work with girls also brought into the youth service groups of young women who had traditionally rejected such provision, (for example, young lesbians) or those who had been forbidden to attend mixed provision. In this way connections could be made between a range of issues such as gender, race, disability and sexuality and how ideas about these impinge on the lives of young people.

Interest in using these ideas in youth work with young men has developed in recent years (Lloyd, 1990; Davidson, 1990) but it remains small scale and localized. Gay youth groups are the exception but these remain largely confined to larger cities. It may be the case that the development of peer education will provide a means of building on and extending this aspect of youth work, by taking the focus away from the group itself. In this way young men may feel they have permission to explore sensitive topics, since it is with the aim of helping other young people.

7 Rights and relevance

Introduction

What have we attempted to explore in this book? In Chapter 1 we set out to examine various aspects of young people's development. This review of the psycho-social literature gives considerable insights into how young people move from childhood to adulthood. However we have to be careful not to let this perspective limit our vision by viewing young people as 'proto-adults' with no valid viewpoint or perspective themselves. In Chapter 2 the health issues associated with adolescence were explored. Too often the agenda in health terms is set by adults who problematize youth health. The epidemiological studies described in the first half of this chapter epitomize this approach, by identifying 'problem' issues and attempting to gather data on their frequency or incidence. This gives us little idea of the salience of these issues in young people's lives and only a poor indication (through statistical association) of how different factors combine within young people's overall lifestyles. In contrast to these the chapter ends with a set of illuminative, ethnographic studies which attempt to 'get under the skin' of adolescent life to examine the diversity of ways in which young people experience youth and the attendant health issues. The more holistic pictures these present may offer vital clues for health educators in planning and evaluating interventions aimed at young people.

Chapter 3 focused specifically on the context of the school, attempting to explore the models and paradigms which structure education on health. Here we also explored the concept of empowerment and how this tends to operate at the level of the individual. The strengths and weaknesses of the empowerment model were analysed and it was suggested that the perspective of the young person has often to be sacrificed to the need for schools to operate within a 'safe' and uncontroversial model. Collective, and hence more radical, approaches may present challenges to ways in which other topics are addressed within the school.

We went on, in the next chapter, to explore the problems of trying to deliver education on health from the perspective of the educator within the school setting. Conflicts in government policy, professional training issues, lack of managerial support, and the barriers to communication with parents and young people are among the issues which we consider.

In Chapter 5, having recognized that health education within schools remains problematic, we examined the possibilities within the community for developing forms of health education which cater for the heterogeneity of youth. It was recognized that there may be fewer constraints within youth work than there are in school settings, but a range of difficulties which beset schools are also present to a lesser extent in this arena. In particular, moral and ethical issues (whether real or imagined) may inhibit workers from addressing certain areas deemed to be sensitive or controversial. However it may be the case that community-based approaches offer more potential to develop strategies for effective work with young people. The dangers of 'hit and run' campaigns, however, which take little account of the contested nature of much health education, are also highlighted.

Chapter 6 examined some of these alternative approaches in the community more closely. The theme of 'marrying' young people's perspective with that of the programme planners was developed. At the same time recognition of the impact of structural factors on young people's lives demands that health educators recognize the diversity of opportunities and constraints on how young people understand and perceive health in their lives.

Through the course of this book we have seen how a number of issues concerning young people's health and adult professional approaches to health education in school and communities contain conflicts or even paradoxes. Thus, for example, we have looked at the disparity between young people's knowledge of health issues and their actual behaviours. We have often alluded to young people's perceived invulnerability and their subsequent risk behaviours. We have explored the intention of teachers to develop health education in a holistic way and then compared this with the constraints, real or imagined, surrounding teacher and school approaches to health education. We have speculated on the potential of community education approaches but have also been forced to acknowledge their limitations built as they are around a network of volunteers, both adolescent and adult. Underlying all these issues is the question of how we can integrate genuine adult concerns for young people's health with young people's own priorities and perspectives on health.

As we have seen in this book, therefore, a considerable amount of attention has been paid by adult society generally, and health professionals in particular, to the subject of health interventions on behalf of young people and on the need to provide specialist services or advice for them. Laudable and welcome though this focus is, many policies concerning health issues are formulated on the basis of adult assumptions about what services or information young people might need.

On the whole, agendas are still set by well-meaning adults who feel they have the wisdom and experience of their years and their personal and professional experience to help them decide what is best for young people. Others would maintain that a more sinister rationale is at work, and would maintain that 'doing our best for young people' can often be interpreted as an unconscious but pervasive way of maintaining social control over a cohort that is often seen as threatening and subversive (Apple, 1979; Jones and Wallace, 1992; Griffin, 1993). Cultural theory (van Gennep, 1960) stresses that having excluded young people and provoked risk-taking

181

behaviours by this exclusion, adult society is also likely to use their 'at risk' status to attempt to control their actions. Can we take account of the young person's perspective without the imposition of social control?

The main thrust of this book therefore has been a consideration of school and community approaches to health education for young people and a drawing out of an emphasis on the need to consider young people's own views. Tilford (1992) noted that young people's own views of their health concerns do not entirely equate with those of adults and she pointed to the work of Balding (1987) and Friedman (1989) in support of her argument. If we believe that health agendas set by adults differ considerably from those felt to be appropriate by young people themselves, we need to address this anomaly.

In addition to emphasizing that health education must be founded around topics that are actually of salience to young people, we would also suggest that health educators need to use *methods* which understand and genuinely respect adolescent interests. Teachers and other educators might best contribute to the learning process by encouraging and supporting activities and learning experiences which enhance the self-esteem and self-efficacy of young people. This would influence teaching approaches in health education in making them less didactic, by allowing time and space for reflection and discussion, and by encouraging self-agency in adolescence. In addition, the death of didacticism and the development of a more reflective approach might allow us to take account of the 'mythologies' about health still held by young people.

Much of the present authors' concerns centre around the inability of health education to match young people's own concerns in ways which engage their interest and have an impact on their behaviour. These concerns arise from the empirical observations carried out through a variety of project settings in the last twelve years. During this period we have also identified two further trends which we think worthy of comment in this final chapter. The first concerns the issue of children's 'rights', and we explore this in the section which follows. The second concerns the growing 'professionalization' of health education and the extent to which this has been accompanied by a deskilling of parent roles in the health education of young people.

Young people's rights

Concern over children's rights has been brought sharply into focus in recent years on an international scale. From concern over child abuse by rock stars to debates over the rights of young people to divorce parents they deem to be unsatisfactory, the tabloid press has been fascinated by certain aspects of this issue but notably silent in relation to others. The introduction of the Children Act in England in 1989 (HMSO, 1989) and pressure at a political level for a wide range of legislation can be seen in relation to wider societal themes. Thus over the last fifteen years we have seen the development of consumerism and the establishment of the primacy of the market place. It has also occurred at a time when the behaviour of young people has come under increasing scrutiny by policy-makers and researchers, and when, despite an overt focus on specific sorts of children's rights being enshrined and protected in law, there has been an erosion of the autonomy and depletion of other rights, particularly in the UK and USA.

The 'rights' debate has also taken place within a climate where the category of 'youth' (particularly working-class and black youth) has re-emerged as a focus of moral panic on both sides of the Atlantic. Within these broader questions debates over the health rights of young people highlight some of the contradictions and paradoxes inherent within the concept of children's rights.

The 'rights' approach has received a certain degree of criticism from some social scientists and professionals working with young people (Frost and Stein, 1989; Walton, 1994). Part of the resistance to the notion lies in the fact that the 'rights' issue inevitably draws attention to the disempowered state of young people *generally* (assuming a degree of homogeneity of

183

experience and interests related to age), and away from the particularly disempowered state of certain categories of young people. In other words, though youth is a disadvantaging factor, poverty, race and gender may be structurally more important in determining life chances and health behaviour and outcomes. The focus on 'youth' as a category distracts from an understanding of this. Frost and Stein (1992) for example argue that:

> Young people experience powerlessness through their status as young people – by exclusion from decision making processes, for example, in schools, or on a wider basis, by their exclusion from the political process. However this powerlessness is overlaid by other categories, most notably social class, disability, ethnicity and gender which interact with generation to produce a matrix of power and powerlessness. (Frost and Stein, 1992, p.162)

Chisholm and du Bois-Raymond (1993) in studying youth in a European context, similarly argue that the transitions from youth to adulthood are complex, fragmented and heavily influenced by systematic social inequalities. This perspective is gaining more acceptance by researchers into youth in recent years but has tended to be neglected in favour of an emphasis on developmental concerns in much previous study.

The framing of the legislation on rights also emphasizes and prioritizes the rights of the individual. While this may be appropriate within the context of existing legal frameworks, many of the issues identified within the charter itself demand collective action organization. Issues facing young people in care, the young homeless, child prostitutes, or the young gay targets of homophobic attacks for instance may demand concerted action at a political level which goes way beyond the notion of asserting the rights of the individual.

At a policy level, the adoption of the UN Convention on the Rights of the Child by the General Assembly of the United Nations in 1991 has had a powerful impact on the 123 countries which have agreed to ratify it. Signatories agree to be legally bound by the Convention and to report regularly on the progress being made towards achievement of the provisions within the charter. However countries are permitted under certain conditions to submit reservations and declarations to particular aspects with which they are unable or unwilling to comply. Clearly these caveats can permit skilful manipulation to allow for maximum publicity and little action on the substance. In the UK the Children's Rights Development Unit was set up to draw together a National Agenda for Children which includes a set of minimum standards for children and young people's civil, political, economic, social and cultural rights (CRDU, 1994).

It remains unclear how the unit will organize training for professionals, how young people themselves will be drawn into consultation and on precisely which issues the agenda will focus. In fact the UK has recently been strongly criticized by the UN monitoring committee. Despite intensive lobbying by civil servants, the committee produced a report highly critical of British governmental 'lynch pin' strategies for dealing with youth, particularly in relation to plans to introduce secure training centres for 12- to 14-year-olds, and to aspects of the treatment of child refugees. The high level of child poverty attributed to changes in social security regulations was also noted (Travis, in the *Guardian*, 28 January 1995, p.4). Thus the convention is able to adopt a lobbying role in relation to member countries but it remains to be seen if this will be effective and whether it will enable or encourage reform on other levels.

Nevertheless, it is clear that however well co-ordinated and well intentioned such a movement may be at a policy level, there are powerful paradoxes inherent in the concept of children's rights. Walton (1995) argues, for instance, that it is essentially a paternalistic strategy offering to define and frame rights on behalf of, rather than with, young people. That the movement fails to engage with youth cultures is clear and it may in fact, be dissonant with currents such as 'the right to party' and the 'hedonism for hard times' suggested by Redhead and other commentators on rave culture (Redhead, 1993).

185

It is clear that young people themselves are not only inactive in the children's rights movement in terms of defining and asserting their rights, but are in effect actually excluded from this process. The initiation of *Who Cares?* a self-help group for young people leaving care represents one attempt to organize around an agenda which includes children's rights in the broadest sense but it is woefully unsupported by the existence of other pressure groups for young people's issues.

Despite the overt attention paid to young people's rights, however, there are broader social forces currently at work which run counter to the policy thrust embodied in the children's charter. Davies (1986), among others, has highlighted the ways in which 'the condition of youth' has often been used as a barometer of the social ills of the wider society. When times are troubled and there is a high level of economic and social uncertainty, young people are seized upon and held up as a symptom of what is going wrong. However, they also get caught up in a scapegoating process whereby they are somehow also to blame for social, moral and even economic decline. Recent attempts in both the USA and the UK (Griffin, 1993) to blame young single mothers for the decline of family values and the breakdown of the fabric of society at large represent a good case of this syndrome, as western governments seek to balance spending on welfare commitments in a period when the demands on the system set by a growing proportion of elderly people are bound to increase.

Young people are not seen within the welfare system as having the potential to exercise considered judgement or autonomy. Thus 16-year-olds in the UK, whatever their circumstances, have no entitlement to social security support. It is envisaged that forcing families to assume responsibility for young people into their twenties will both transform 'family' values and relieve the state of responsibility for social policy in relation to the young.

Thus the children's rights movement would seem in theory to provide a mechanism for highlighting inequalities and issues facing children but it is limited in reality in being able to

186

provide a framework for exploring the hidden or unstated concerns of young people. Frost and Stein (1989) argue for a focus on 'empowerment' rather than rights. Although this word has been overused in the literature on youth and community, it is useful in bringing the notion of power into the debate. In this sense, themes and changes in, for example, power relationships within families can be identified at a micro-level while broader themes of change in family structure and dynamics can be addressed. As a number of critics have noted, despite the much vaunted concern about the decline of family standards and values, little social research has been undertaken in relation to how young people interact with families after early childhood and in particular how families help or hinder the development of viable identities (Brannen *et al.*, 1994; Jones and Wallace, 1992; Griffin, 1993).

Jones and Wallace (1992) argue that the concept of 'citizenship' allows for an understanding of youth which includes both the private and the public aspects of growing up. They further suggest that it brings together the notion of the rights and the obligations of adults to young people. Thus both developmental and structural aspects of the youth process can be identified and accommodated within this framework. There are clear problems with this scheme which Jones and Wallace acknowledge. To what extent, for example, can young people be citizens without being economically dependent? Moreover is it not the case that the 'rights' of the child in the setting of the nuclear family are only 'third party' rights, administered by the parent on behalf of the young person? To what extent does this represent real independence?

Jones and Wallace also debunk the 'consumerist' interpretation of rights. This most recent (in the UK) manifestation of citizenship in public debate emphasizes power through choice in the consumer market. The incomes of most young people, however, are so low that after essential needs have been met, young people have little left with which to exercise their choice or rights as consumers. They are cruelly disadvantaged if this

187

is to be our modern definition of the exercise of the rights of the individual.

In this section we have looked at the broader development of ideas about young people's rights. A worldwide impetus to transform the condition of young people by giving them a set of inalienable rights is, however, as we have seen, too easily used to distract attention away from other structural inequalities that may be more alienating or disadvantaging than youth itself. Then, too, the emphasis on individual rights may make it difficult to exercise the sort of collective action which could lobby for change of some of these structural conditions.

Traditionally children, as dependents of their parents, have had their rights by proxy, mediated by the stewardship of their parents. Some writers have seen the emphasis on the individual young person's rights (independent of the family) as a convenient tool with which to attack or undermine the influence of families seen to be 'poor' or 'bad' (Walton, 1994). If this is indeed the case, then it is markedly ineffective as the UK government swings from general statements blaming families for social problems to specific policies which force young people back into dependence on those families for longer periods of their life.

We turn in this next section to the question of how these broad reflections on the questions of young people's rights are expressed in the arena of health education and advice for young people.

Young people's rights to health education and information

When we move away from this broader debate to the specific case of young people's rights to ask for and receive appropriate health advice and education, we enter a minefield through which a variety of professionals have been gingerly picking their way for at least a decade and a half. For, moving from the abstract notion of children's rights to be treated as individuals to these specifics brings us into the contested ground where parents feel they have a right to exercise their authority for the benefit and welfare of young people who are still dependent on them. Nowhere has this been clearer than in the realm of education about sexual behaviour and in the provision of services to meet young people's sexual needs. The literature increasingly reflects this sense of children having the right to be educated on matters like sexuality, drug misuse and so on, and we have explored in earlier chapters how such matters are now seen as appropriate for inclusion in the curriculum. Does the formalization of such education, however, deny children the right to be educated with respect to their personal development and maturity? We ask this question merely to explore the paradox that, in order to improve the level and type of health education for all young people, we may be forced by the structures in place in schools to deprive individuals of their right to be educated when they are ready and able to take advantage of it. To illustrate this point we might look at the very different rates at which young people achieve sexual maturity. At what point does it become appropriate to stop talking about sexuality in an abstract or biological sense and to start talking to young men and women as if this represented an area of experience with which they were familiar and in which they might be facing personal challenges and problems? Inappropriately pitched education on these issues is at best wasted and meaningless, and at worst potentially harmful if it normalizes a state of affairs which is not normal for that young person.

Ideally we might as educators like to treat each young person as an individual, to give each child the appropriate knowledge and guidance at the point when it is required. The educational system does not have this luxury and the only people who do – parents – seem only too keen to have their role stripped from them in many spheres of health education by the growing 'professionalization' of health education. Frankham (1993), reporting an interview study with the parents of teenagers, notes:

> Parents justify their reticence to talk about sex [...] as a desire not to give information that their children are not ready for. Many of

189

them judge 'readiness' in terms of the sorts of relationships they feel their children are having and common was the confident expression that their children were not involved or ready for 'that sort of (sexual) relationship' yet. What they seem to fear is some sort of curtailment of their child's innocence.

(Frankham, 1993, p.27)

Do the attempts to raise the standard of teaching and learning on health by the education professions have a perverse effect on parents' perceived ability to take on the task themselves? Are parents, in fact, 'deskilled', by the development of formal curricula and innovative teaching methods? There is some evidence that this is indeed the case (Young, 1991). Young's survey revealed that parents are as bamboozled by schemes that talk about health-promoting schools as they are by schemes that aim to introduce new teaching methods in maths.

There is, of course, a rather 'chicken and egg' side to this argument. Has health education become formalized in schools as a result of the inability of parents to guide and help their children to develop appropriately in this sphere? Or has the growth of health education as a specialist curricular area edged parents out from a role which they may have performed reasonably well, albeit somewhat intuitively? The evidence is mixed and the jury may well have to stay out on this one.

What seems clear is that many parents do want schools and other education agencies to take on an interventionist role in respect of their children's health education, especially in certain spheres (Wyness, 1992). Frankham *et al.*'s study (1992), for instance, makes it clear that it is often so difficult for parents to acknowledge either their own or their older child's sexuality, because of the nature of family relationships, that in many cases it is easier for an 'outsider' to step in and take over the discussion of difficult issues. Despite some well-publicized episodes, however, of sex education startling parents into an acknowledgement of what is going on in class-rooms and exciting a vociferous minority into an agitated state, most parents are keen for schools to tackle these issues, and feel that it is an appropriate part of their child's educational experience (Young, 1994).

The assumption by teachers and others of this mantle, however, makes it too easy to feel that learning is only accomplished through formal instruction or staged dialogues. Whatever inputs children get formally from school on health issues, they are continually schooled by their parents through role modelling, through informal discussion and comment on neighbourhood affairs and personalities, through incidental commentaries on the stories in soap operas and so on. It is these everyday interactions that cement together the blocks of information or the discussion exercises that schools provide, and neither party to this process seems well enough tuned in to regard this process and to acknowledge its importance, despite the evidence that these settings are the most effective in transmitting values and in contextualizing information (Prendergast and Prout, 1987). Farquhar (1990), for instance, found that the main source of 8- and 10-year-old children's beliefs about HIV/AIDS was the media and discussions with parents. Older children demonstrate their changing relationship with their parents by seeking broader sources of information and advice on different topics (the peer group or teen magazines), but Allen (1987), for example, still found among her sample of teenage girls in three English cities that mothers were a preferred source of information and advice on many health-related topics.

We must be careful that we do not diminish this relationship by the overprofessionalization of health teaching in educational settings, for there are considerations beyond those of the most efficient transmission of 'correct' knowledge. Farrell (1978), Fox and Inazu (1980) and Bury (1984), for instance, all found that good parent-child communication (particularly mother-daughter communication) had positive outcomes in terms of adolescents' later sexual behaviour.

We would do well as educators, therefore, to resist the temptation to take on too much of the responsibility for children's health education. A wiser course may be to accept the role and

191

value of parent-child interactions in shaping young people's beliefs and behaviours and to work to strengthen that influence by developing closer partnership with parents. Such a task is easier to say than to do.

Many professional educators do worry about the extent to which they stand *in loco parentis*, as we have seen in Chapter 4. Both parties in a sense need reassurance that there is a consensual agenda on health and about the methods which should be used to promote it. Yet few schools or other educational agencies seem to have the appropriate mechanisms which would facilitate dialogue and develop consensus. Schools now have very clear directives from central government to consult with the parent body, both through developing formal levels of participation (school governors, or school boards in Scotland), and through less formal channels. Scottish schools, for instance, in a drive to improve their overall effectiveness are encouraged to consult parents by questionnaire as part of a programme for measuring and evaluating the ethos of the school.

Such developments can establish the principle of participation, but there is little evidence in reality of the true development of 'voice' with the consumers of the educational process. Even where determined attempts are made to consult parents the process is skewed towards the well-educated parents with the vocabulary and grammar, the social confidence to make a point at an open meeting and the social equipment to deal in agendas and minutes. Clearly this is a problem which confronts the whole of the education system, not just health education, but it can be more acute in this arena. Young (1991), for instance, describes a programme, one aim of which was to increase the level of parental understanding and collaboration in health education. Commenting on the low levels of parent understanding and interest he concludes that in order to engage parents' interest 'it may be necessary to consider a flexible component on the details of the curriculum which each individual school could insert in the parents' guide reflecting local community issues' (Young, 1991, p.229). Such a statement would be almost inconceivable in the context of the mathematics curriculum or the English course. Schools do not have the experience and skills to develop or feel comfortable with a dialogue whose appropriateness is not accepted in many spheres of the curriculum. Nor also do the majority of parents have the practice, the skills and the experience to make their views felt in this sort of debate.

Young people learning about health

It is clear from the preceding chapters that there is a need for more attention to be paid to the affective and social aspects of adolescent development in designing programmes in health education. A genuine view of adolescents in the role of 'learners concerned with social and personal selves' is needed. Pintrich *et al.* (1993) have argued that theories of conceptual change which ignore motivation and intentions do not adequately cover adolescent learning. Boekaerts (1992 and 1993) has also developed a theoretical account of the relationship between motivation and learning, taking into account seriously the subjective experiences of the learner. This drives home the point that teachers and other health educators, who ignore learners' understandings of, and feelings about, the nature and significance of learning tasks, are likely to find a fundamental lack of agreement between their own and their pupils' conceptions of health issues. There is clearly a possible threat to learning if teachers and other health educators act as if young people were simply learning systems capable of solving problems. Such a stance may function as an obscuring filter through which health knowledge and the social behavioural skills young people need to learn – and the relationship between prior and new knowledge – are not well integrated. Thus we would want to propose that the perspective which best accords with the 'learning self' in young people is essentially social and affective. This may be seen as a classic recipe for curricular design in health education, but the wider issue here is about the need for the content and methods of health education to reflect the changing social paradigm in which young people operate.

Much of health education is still based on a rationalist view of social conduct, as we have shown in Chapter 3. But young people live their lives today in a post-modernist consumer culture, characterized in part by an expectation that needs and desires can be gratified through purchase of different commodities. Thus health education tends to emphasize an ethic which is rationalist and almost Presbyterian in its insistence on rewards and punishments for good and bad living. Youth culture on the other hand, driven by the power of advertising, emphasizes the pleasure principle and legitimizes the seeking of instant gratification. Young people find the message of 'live now, pay later' as attractive in health terms as they do in terms of paying for their consumer purchases.

Life in the past could be interpreted much more as a 'package' deal. Then, given certain structural conditions, like class and gender, the expectation was that young people would acquire a fairly narrow set of values which 'limited' their behaviour (Bourdieu, 1984). Increasingly, as society has become more affluent and the old social mores relating to age, class and gender have broken down, individuals are freer to 'appropriate' meanings into their lives from wherever they choose, except for those young people who are denied access to consumer culture and live in relative poverty.

Throughout the book we have noted several examples of transformational leisure activities of young people. By using alcohol, other drugs, driving fast cars or attending all-night raves, young people can accomplish a move from the everyday world to a hedonistic leisure sphere. The pattern of activities may be different for different groups of young people yet such diversification and individualization of style and of choice of activities fits in very well with views of post-modernism. Health education has to try a lot harder to understand and incorporate the pleasure principle if it is to match with young people's own agendas.

Final comment

Within the preceding chapters of this book we have touched on many difficult issues for health professionals to debate and emphasized the problems involved in linking young people's perspectives with the concerns of adult society. In so doing we have probably raised more questions than we have answered. If this book has done nothing more than bring into focus these issues for further debate we are happy. If we believe in the empowerment of adolescents and in their right to learn about and control their own health then it is important that health education attempts to meet the needs of the *real* lives that young people are living today.

Bibliography

Aaro, L.E., Wold, B., Kannas, L. and Rimpela, M. (1986) 'Health behaviour in school-children. A WHO cross-national survey, *Health Promotion*, 1, 1, pp.17–33.

Abbott, R. (1994) Learning Makes Sense: Recreating Education for a Changing Future. London, Education 2,000.

Abel, T. and McQueen, D. (1992) 'The formation of health lifestyles: A new empirical concept'. Paper presented to the BSA and ESMS Joint Conference on Health in Europe, Edinburgh, 18–21 September 1992.

Abrams, D., Abraham, C., Spears, R. and Harks, D. (1990) 'AIDS invulnerability: Relationships, sexual behaviour and attitudes amongst 16–19 year olds', in Aggleton, P., Davies, P. and Hart, G. (eds) *AIDS: Individual, Cultural and Policy Dimensions*. London, Falmer Press.

Aggleton, P. (1989) 'Evaluating health education about AIDS', in Aggleton, P., Hart, G. and Davies, P. (eds) *AIDS: Social Representations, Social Practices*. London, Falmer Press.

Aggleton, P. and Homans, H. (eds) (1988) *Social Aspects of AIDS*. London, Falmer Press.

Aggleton, P., Toft, M. and Warwick, I. (1992) 'Working for young people: priorities for HIV/AIDS health promotion in local settings', in Evans, B., Sandberg, S. and Watson, S. (eds) *Working Where the Risks Are: Issues in HIV Prevention*. London, Health Education Authority.

Aggleton, P., Weeks, J. and Taylor-Laybourn, M. (1993) 'Voluntary sector responses to HIV and AIDS: A framework for analysis', in Aggleton, P., Davies, P., Hart, G. (eds) *Social Aspects of AIDS: Facing the Second Decade*. London, Falmer.

Ajzen, I. and Fishbein, M. (1980) *Understanding Attitudes and Predicting Behaviour*. Englewood Cliffs, NJ, Prentice-Hall.

Allen, I. (1987) *Education in Sex and Personal Relationships*. London, Policy Studies Institute Research Report No. 665.

Allen, I. (1991) *Family Planning and Pregnancy Counselling Projects for Young People*. London, Policy Studies Institute.

Almond, L. (1983) 'A guide to practice', *British Journal of Physical Education*, 14, 5, pp.134–35.

197

Altman, D. (1993) 'Expertise, Legitimacy and the Centrality of Community', in Aggleton, P., Davies, P. and Hart, G. (eds) *AIDS: Facing the Second Decade*. London, Falmer.

Apple, M.W. (1979) *Ideology and Curriculum*. London, Routledge and Kegan Paul.

Arborelius, E. and Bremberg, S. (1988) 'It is *your* decision! – Behavioural effects of a student-centred health education model at school for adolescents', *Journal of Adolescence*, **11**, pp.287–97.

Arkin, A. (1993) 'How to meet the need for dialogue', *Times Educational Supplement*, 29 January 1993, p.6.

Ashton, M. (ed.) (1991) *Drug Misuse in Britain. National Audit of Drug Misuse Statistics*. London, ISDD.

Association of Metropolitan Authorities (AMA) (1993) *Local Authorities and Community Development. A Strategic Opportunity for the 1990s*. London, Association of Metropolitan Authorities.

Backett, K. and Alexander, H. (1989) 'What does health mean to children?' Working paper (unpublished). Edinburgh, Research Unit in Health and Behavioural Change.

Bagnall, G. (1989) 'Alcohol education for 13 year olds: Does it work?' *British Journal of Addictions*, **85**, pp.150–70.

Balding, J. (1986) 'Mayfly. A study of 1,237 pupils aged 14–15 who completed the Health Related Behaviour Questionnaire in May 1988'. Unpublished report, HEA Schools Health Education Unit, School of Education, University of Exeter.

Balding, J. (1987) *Young People in 1986*, Exeter, HEA Schools Health Education Unit, University of Exeter.

Bandura, A. (1977) *Social Learning Theory*. Englewood Cliffs, NJ, Prentice Hall.

Bandura, A. (1981) 'Self-referent thought: A developmental analysis of self-efficacy', in Flavell, J.H. and Ross, L. (eds) *Social Cognitive Development*. Cambridge, Cambridge University Press.

Bandura, A. (1986) *Social Foundation of Thought and Action*. Englewood Cliffs, NJ, Prentice Hall.

Barnes, G. (1977) 'The development of adolescent drinking behaviour: An evaluative review of the impact of the socialisation process within the family', *Adolescence*, **12**, pp.571–91.

Baron, J. and Brown, R.V. (eds) (1991) *Teaching Decision Making to Adolescents*. Hillsdale, NJ, Lawrence Erlbaum Associates.

Barrigan, S. (1993) 'Sky High Bananas', *Youth and Policy*, **43**, pp.67–75.

Becker, M.H. (ed) (1984) *The Health Belief Model and Personal Health Behaviour*. New Jersey, Charles B Slack, Thorofare.

Bell, A. (1991) 'Growing up Gay', *Scottish Child*, November, pp. 14–17.

Bellaby, P. (1990) 'To risk or not to risk? Uses and limitations of Mary

Douglas on risk-acceptability for understanding health and safety at work and road accidents', *Sociological Review*, 38, 3, pp.456–83.

Bellingham, K. and Gillies, P. (1993) 'Evaluation of an AIDS programme for young adults', *Journal of Epidemiology and Health*, 47, pp.134–38.

Biggs, S.J. Bender, M. and Foreman, J. (1983) 'Are there psychological differences between persistent solvent abusing delinquents and delinquents who do not use solvents', *British Journal of Adolescence*, 6, pp.71–86.

Blaxter, M. (1987) 'Alcohol consumption', in Cox, B.D. (ed) *The Health and Lifestyle Survey*. Cambridge, The Health Promotion Research Trust.

Blaxter, M. (1990) *Health and Lifestyles*. London, Routledge.

Boekaerts, M. (1993) 'Being concerned with well-being and with learning', *Educational Psychologist*, 28, 2, pp.149–67.

Boekaerts, M. (1993) 'The adaptable learning process: initiating and maintaining behavioural change', *Applied Psychology: an International Review*, 41; pp.337–97.

Boskind-White, M. and White, W.C. (1987) *Bulimarexia: The Binge/Purge Cycle*, 2nd edn. New York and London, Norton.

Bosma, H.A. (1992) 'Identity in adolescence: Managing commitments', in Adams, G.R., Gullotta, T. and Montemayor R. (eds) *Identity Formation During Adolescence*. Newbury Park, Sage.

Bourdieu, P. (1984) *Distinction: A Social Critique of the Judgement of Taste*, London, Routledge.

Bowie, C. and Ford, N. (1989) 'Sexual behaviour of young people and the risk of HIV infection' *Journal of Epidemiology and Community Health*, 43, pp.61–5.

Brake, M. (1980) *The Sociology of Youth Culture*, London, Routledge and Kegan Paul.

Brannen, J., Dodd, K., Oakley, A. and Storey, P. (1994) *Young People, Health and Family Life*. Buckingham, Open University Press.

Bridges Project (1988) *Fizz, Fat and Fasting*. Edinburgh, Bridges Project.

British Market Research Bureau (1990) *Youth Lifestyles 1990*. London, Mintel Publications Ltd.

Bury, J. (1984) *Teenage Pregnancy in Britain*. London, Birth Control Trust.

Bury, J. (1991) 'Teenager social behaviour and the impact of AIDS', *Health Education Journal*, 50, 1, pp.43–8.

Children's Rights Development Unit (CRDU) (1994a) 'The United Nations' convention of the rights of the child: Briefing papers'. London, CRDU.

Children's Rights Development Unit (CRDU) (1994b) 'Scottish Agenda for Children'. Draft agenda, Glasgow, Scottish Child Law Centre.

Chisholm, L. and Du Bois-Raymond, N. (1993) 'Youth transitions, gender and social change', *Sociology*, 27, 2, pp.259–79.

Clausen, J.A. (1975) 'The social meaning of differential physical and sexual maturation', in Dragastin, S. and Elder, G. (eds) *Adolescence in the Life Cycle*. New York, John Wiley.

Clements, I. and Buczkiewicz, M. (1993) *Approaches to Peer Led Health Education*, London, Health Education Authority.

Clift, S., Stears, D., Legg, S., Memon, A. and Ryan, L. (1989) *The HIV/AIDS Education and Young People Project: Report on Phase One*. Canterbury, HIV/AIDS Education Research Unit, Department of Educational Studies, Christ Church College.

Coffield, F. (1992) 'Young people and illicit drugs'. Summary research report, Northern Regional Health Authority and Durham University.

Coffield, F., Borrill, C. and Marshall, S. (1986) *Growing Up at the Margins*. Milton Keynes, Open University Press.

Coffield, F. and Gofton, L. (1994) *Drugs and Young People*. London, Institute for Public Policy Research.

Coggans, N., Shewan, D., Henderson, M. and Davies, J.B. (1991a) 'The impact of school-based drug education', *British Journal of Addiction*, 86, 1099–109.

Coggans, N., Shewan, D., Henderson, M., and Davies, J.B. (1991b) 'Could do better – an evaluation of drug education' *Druglink*, September/October, pp.14–16.

Coggans, N., Shewan, D., Henderson, M., Davies, J.B. and O'Hagan, F. (1990) *National Evaluation of Drug Education in Scotland. Final Report*. Edinburgh, Scottish Education Department.

Cohen, S. (1972) *Moral Panics and Folk Devils*. London, MacGibbon and Kee.

Cohen, S. (1973) 'The volatile solvents', *Public Health Review*, 2, 2, pp.185–214.

Coleman, J.C. (1979) 'Current view of the adolescent process', in Coleman, J.C. (ed) *The School Years*. London, Methuen.

Coleman, J.C. and Coleman, E.Z. (1984) 'Adolescent attitudes to authority', *Journal of Adolescence*, 7, pp.131–41.

Coleman, J.C. and Hendry, L.B. (1990) *The Nature of Adolescence*, 2nd edn. London and New York, Routledge.

Coleman, J.C. and Warren-Adamson, C. (eds) (1992) *Youth Policy in the 1990s*. London, Routledge.

Conger, J.T. and Petersen, A.C. (1984) *Adolescence and Youth*, New York, Harper and Row.

Conley, J. (1978) 'Health education comes of age', *Monitor*, 54, pp.4–5.

Csikszentmihalyi, M. (1975) *Beyond Boredom and Anxiety*. San Francisco, Jossey-Bass.

Csikszentmihalyi, M. and Larson, R. (1984) *Being Adolescent: Conflict*

200

and Growth in the Teenage Years. New York, Basic Books.

Currie, C., McQueen, D.V. and Tyrell, H. (1987) The First Year of the RUHBC/SHEG/WHO Survey of Health Behaviours of Scottish Schoolchildren, Edinburgh, RUHBC.

Damon, W. (1983) Social and Personality Development: Infancy through Adolescence. New York, Norton.

Davidson, N. (1990) Boys will Be ...? Sex education and Young Men. London, Bedford Press.

Davies, B. (1977) 'Attitudes towards school among early and late maturing adolescent girls', Journal of Genetic Psychology, 131, pp.261–66.

Davies, B. (1986) Threatening Youth: Towards a National Youth Policy. Milton Keynes, Open University Press.

Davies, E. and Furnham, A. (1986) 'Body satisfaction in adolescent girls', British Journal of Medical Psychology, 59, 3, pp. 279–88.

Davies, J. and Coggans, N. (1991) The Facts About Adolescent Drug Abuse. London, Cassell.

Davis, J. (1990) Youth and the Condition of Britain: Images of Adolescent Conflict. London, Athlone Press.

Deem, R. (1989) 'Feminism and leisure studies: Opening up new directions', in Wimbush, E. and Talbot, M. (eds) Relative Freedoms: Women and Leisure. Milton Keynes, Open University Press.

Department for Education (DfE) (1993) 'Sex Education in Schools: Proposed Revision of Circular 11/87. London, Department for Education.

Department of Education and Science (DES) (1991) The Education (National Curriculum) Attainment Targets and Programmes of Study in Science Order. London, HMSO.

Department of Health (DoH) (1992) The Health of the Nation. White Paper. London, HMSO.

Department of Health (DoH) (1993) The Health of the Nation, Key Area Handbook: HIV/AIDS and Sexual Health, London, Department of Health.

Devereux, E.C. (1976) 'Backyard versus little league baseball: The impoverishment of children's play', in Landers, D. (ed.) Social Problems in Athletics. Illinois, University of Illinois Press.

Devine, M., Black, H. and Gray, D. (1993) Health Education in Scottish Schools, Edinburgh, Scottish Council for Research in Education.

Dick, S. (1994) The Peer Education Project on Sexual Health at Trinity Academy 1990–93: An Evaluative Study. Edinburgh, Brook Advisory Service.

Donoghue, J. (1991) 'Health Education and the national curriculum', Health Education Journal, 50, 1, pp.16–17.

Dorn, N. (1983) Alcohol, Youth and the State, Oxford, Croom Helm.

Dowsett, G., Davis, M. and Connell, B. (1992) 'Gay men, HIV/AIDS and

Social Research: An antipodean perspective', in Aggleton, P., Davies, P. and Hart, G. (eds) *AIDS: Rights, Risk and Reason*. London, Falmer.

Dudley, E. (1993) *The Critical Villager: Beyond Community Participation*, London, Routledge.

Eachus, P. (1991) 'Inequalities in health: Locus of control as a radiating factor', *Journal of the Institute of Health Education*, **29**, 2, pp.60–7.

Elias, M.J. (1990) 'The role of affect and social relationships in health behaviour and school health curriculum and instruction', *Journal of School Health*, **60**, 4, pp.157–63.

Elkind, D. (1984) 'Teenage thinking: implications for health care', *Paediatric Nursing*, **10**, pp.383–85.

Elkind, D. (1985) 'Cognitive development and adolescent disabilities', *Journal of Adolescent Health Care*, **6**, pp.84–9.

Emler, N. (1984) 'Differential involvement in delinquency: Towards an interpretation in terms of reputation management', *Progress in Experimental Personality Research*, **13**, pp.173–239.

Epstein, D. (1993) 'Sexual subjects: Some methodological problems in researching sexuality in schools'. Paper given at the Australian Association for Research in Education Conference, 25–27 November.

Epstein, D. (1994) *Challenging Lesbian and Gay Inequalities in Education*. Buckingham, Open University Press.

Erikson, E. (1968) *Identity: Youth in Crisis*. New York, Norton.

European Sports Charter (1975) *'Sport for All' Charter*, European Sports Ministers' Conference. Brussels, Belgium.

Fairley, J. and Paterson, L. (1995) 'Scottish education and the new managerialism', *Scottish Educational Review*, (forthcoming).

Fairmichael, C. (1992) *Young People's Health Project: An Evaluation*, Belfast, North and West Community Unit of Eastern Health and Social Services Board.

Farley, P. (1991) 'From school to community', in Nutbeam, D., Haglund, B., Farley, P. and Tillgren, P. (eds) *Youth Health Promotion: From Theory to Practice in School and Community*. London, Forbes Publications.

Farquhar, C. (1990) *What Do Primary School Children Know About AIDS?* Working Paper No. 1. London, Thomas Coram Research Unit.

Farrell, C. (1978) *My Mother Said ... The Way Young People Learned About Sex and Birth Control*, London, Routledge and Kegan Paul.

Fast Forward (1992) *Dealing in Diversity*. Annual report. Edinburgh, Fast Forward Lifestyles Limited.

Fast Forward (1994) *Headstrong?* Peer Research Project annual report, Edinburgh, Fast Forward Positive Lifestyles Ltd.

Federation of Community Work Training Groups (FCWTG) (1992) *Training Manual 1*, Sheffield, FCWTG.

Fend, H. (1990) 'Ego-strength development and pattern of social relationships', in Bosma, H.A. and Jackson, A.E. (eds) *Coping and Self-Concept in Adolescence*. Heidelberg, Springer-Verlag.

Fishbein, M. and Ajzen, I. (1985) *Belief, Attitude, Intention and Behaviour: An Introduction to Theory and Research*. Reading, MA, Addison-Wesley.

Fishbein, M. and Middlestadt, A. (1990) 'Using the theory of reasoned action as a framework for understanding and changing AIDS related behaviours', in Mays, V., Albee, G.N. and Schneider, S.F. (eds) *Primary Prevention of AIDS*, New York, Sage.

Fisher, K. and Collins, J. (eds) (1993) *Homelessness, Health, Care and Welfare*. London, Routledge.

Foley, G. (1993) 'The neighbourhood house: Site of struggle, site of learning', *British Journal of Sociology of Education*, 14, 1, pp.21–37.

Ford, N. (1987) 'Research into heterosexual behaviour with implications for the spread of AIDS', *British Journal of Family Planning*, 13, pp.50–4.

Ford, N. and Bowie, C. (1989) 'Urban-rural variations in the level of heterosexual activity of young people', *Area*, 21, 3, pp.237–48.

Ford, N. and Morgan, K. (1989) 'Heterosexual lifestyles of young people in an English city', *Journal of Population and Social Studies*, 1, pp.167–82.

Forth Valley Health Board (1994) *Health-Related Behaviour of Young People in Schools in Central Region, 1993*. Stirling, Directorate of Public Health Medicine, Forth Valley Health Board.

Fox, G.L. and Inazu, J. (1980) 'Patterns and outcomes of mother-daughter communication about sexuality', *Journal of Social Issues*, 36, 1, pp.7–29.

Frankenberg, R. (1966) *Communities in Britain*. Harmondsworth, Penguin.

Frankham, J. (1993) 'Not in front of the children', *Medical Sociology News*, 18, 2, pp.26–31.

Frankham, J., with Maclure, M. and Stronach, I. (1992) *Not Under My Roof: Families Talking About Sex and AIDS*. London, AVERT.

Fraser, A., Gamble, L. and Kennett, P. (1991) 'Into the Pleasuredome', *Druglink*, 6, 6, pp.12–13.

Freire, P. (1972) *The Pedagogy of the Oppressed*. Harmondsworth, Penguin.

French, J. and Adams, L. (1986) 'From analysis to synthesis', *Health Education Journal*, 45, 2, pp.71–4.

Friedman, H. (1989) 'The health of adolescents: Beliefs and behaviour', *Social Science and Medicine*, 29, 3, pp.309–15.

Frost, N. and Stein, M. (1989) *The Politics of Child Welfare*. Brighton, Harvester/Wheatsheaf.

Furnham, A. (1986) 'Social skills training with adolescents and young adults', in Hollin, C.R. and Trower, P. (eds) *Handbook of Social Skills*

203

Training: Applications across the Life-span. Vol 1. Oxford, Pergamon.

Gardner, C. and Sheppard, J. (1989) *Consuming Passion, The Rise of Retail Culture.* London, Unwin Hyman.

Gatherer, A. (1979) *Is Health Education Effective?* London, Health Education Council.

van Gennep, A. (1960) *The Rites of Passage,* translated Vizedom, C.K. and Caffee, G.L. London, Routledge and Kegan Paul (first published in 1908).

Gerstel, C.J., Ferraios, A.J. and Herdt, G. (1989) 'Widening Circles, An Ethnographic profile of a youth group', in Herdt, G. (ed.) *Gay and Lesbian Youth.* New York, Haworth Press.

Gillies, P. (1989) 'Health behaviour and health promotion in youth', in Martin, C. J. and McQueen, D. (eds) *Readings for A New Public Health.* Edinburgh, Edinburgh University Press.

Gilligan, C. (1990) 'Teaching Shakespeare's sister: Notes from the underground of female adolescence', preface to Gilligan, C., Lyons, N.P. and Hanover, T.J. (eds) *Making Connections: The Relational World of Adolescent Girls at Emma Willard School.* Cambridge, MA, Harvard University Press.

Glendinning, A., Love, J., Shucksmith, J. and Hendry, L.B. (1992) 'Adolescence and health inequalities: Extensions to McIntyre and West', *Social Science and Medicine,* 35, 5, pp.679–87.

Goddard, E. (1989) *Smoking among Secondary School Children in 1988.* OPCS Social Survey Division, London, HMSO.

Gofton, L. (1990) 'On the town: Drink and the "new lawlessness"', *Youth and Policy,* 29, pp.33–9.

Goggin, M. (1993) 'Gay and Lesbian Adolescence', in Moore, S. and Rosenthal, D., *Sexuality and Adolescence.* London, Cassell.

Golding, J. (1987) 'Smoking', in Cox, B.D. (ed.) *The Health and Lifestyle Survey.* Cambridge, The Health Promotion Research Trust.

Goodlad, S. and Hirst, B. (1989) *Peer Tutoring: A Guide to Learning by Teaching.* London, Kogan Page.

Grant, G., Ross, J. and Thornton, A. (1994) *Cambuslang Youth Health Project: Interim Report.* July. Glasgow, Inequalities in Health Project, Greater Glasgow Health Promotion Department.

Gray, J.A.M. and Blythe, G.M. (1979) 'The Failures of Health Education', in Atkinson, J. and Dingwall, R. (eds) *Prospects for the National Health.* London, Croom-Helm.

Green, J. and Chapman, A. (1992) 'The British Community Development Project: Lessons for today', *Community Development Journal,* 27, 2, pp.242–58.

Green, L.W. (1984) 'Health education models', in Matarozzo, D. (ed.) *Behavioural Health: A Handbook of Health.* Enhancement and Disease Prevention. New York, John Wiley.

Griffin, C. (1985) *Typical Girls?* London, Routledge and Kegan Paul.

Griffin, C. (1993) *Representations of Youth: The Study of Youth and Adolescence in Britain and America*. Cambridge, Polity Press.

Griffin, T. (ed.) (1992) *Social Trends*, 22. London, HMSO.

Grinder, R.E. (1978) *Adolescence*. 2nd ed. New York, Wiley.

Guy, A. (1991) *AIDS Action Groups: A Report of Young Person and Adult Training Partnerships in AIDS Education for Young People*. South Shields, South Tyneside Health Promotion Unit.

Hamilton, V. (1992) 'HIV/AIDS: A peer education approach', *Youth and Policy*, 36, pp.27–32.

Harris, S. (1990) *Lesbian and Gay Issues in the English Classroom*. Milton Keynes, Open University Press.

Hastings, G.B. and Scott, A.C. (1988) 'The development of AIDS education material for adolescents', *Journal of Health Education*, 26, 4, pp.164–71.

Head, M. (1987) 'Health beliefs in adolescence – perceptions and control', *Health Education Journal*, 46, 3, pp.100–03.

Hein, K., Cohen, M.I. and Mark, A. (1978) 'Age at first intercourse among homeless adolescent females', *Journal of Paediatrics*, 93, pp.147–48.

Hendry, L.B. (1983) *Growing Up and Going Out*. Aberdeen, Aberdeen University Press.

Hendry, L.B., Glendinning, A., Shucksmith, J., Love, J. and Scott, J. (1993a) 'The developmental context of adolescent lifestyles', in Silbereisen, R. and Todt, E. (eds) *Adolescents in Context: The Interplay of Family, School, Peers and Work in Adjustment*. New York, Springer International.

Hendry, L.B. and Raymond, M. (1983) 'Youth unemployment and lifestyles: Some educational considerations', *Scottish Educational Review*, 15, 1, pp.28–40.

Hendry, L.B., Love, J.G., Craik, I. and Mack, J. (1991a) *Measuring the Benefits of Youth Work*. Report to the Scottish Office Education Department. Department of Education, University of Aberdeen.

Hendry, L.B., and Raymond, M. (1986) 'Psychological/sociological aspects of youth unemployment: An interpretative theoretical model', *Journal of Adolescence*, 9, pp.355–66.

Hendry, L.B., Raymond, M. and Stewart, C. (1984) 'Unemployment, school and leisure: An adolescent study', *Leisure Studies*, 3, pp.175–87.

Hendry, L.B. and Shucksmith, J. (1994) 'Adolescents in the UK', in Hurrelmann, K. (ed.) *International Handbook of Adolescence*. London, Greenwood Press.

Hendry, L.B., Shucksmith, J. and Love, J.G. (1989) *Young People's Leisure and Lifestyles. Report of Phase 1 (1985–89)*. Edinburgh, The

Scottish Sports Council.

Hendry, L.B., Shucksmith, J., Love, J.G., and Glendinning, A. (1993b) *Young People's Leisure and Lifestyles*. London, Routledge.

Hendry, L.B., Shucksmith, J., Philip, K. and Jones, L. (1991b) *Working with Young People on Drugs and HIV in Grampian Region*. Report of a research project for Grampian Health Board. University of Aberdeen, Department of Education.

Hendry, L.B. and Singer, F.E. (1981) 'Sport and the adolescent girl: A case study of one comprehensive school', *Scottish Journal of Physical Education*, 9, 2, pp.19–29.

Henley Centre (1988 and 1989) *Planning for Social Change*. London, The Henley Centre for Forecasting Ltd.

Hirschman, A.O. (1970) *Exit, Voice and Loyalty – Responses to Decline in Firms, Organisations and States*. Harvard, Harvard University Press.

HMSO (1959) *The Youth Service in England and Wales*. [The Albemarle Report]. London, HMSO.

HMSO (1989) *The Children and Young Persons Act*. London, HMSO.

HMSO (1991) *Youth Work in Scotland: A Report by HM Inspectors of Schools*. Edinburgh, HMSO.

HMSO (1993) *Aids and Drug Misuse Update*. Report by the Advisory Council on the Misuse of Drugs. Edinburgh, HMSO.

Holland, J., Ramazonoglu, C. and Scott, S. (1990a) *Sex, Risk and Danger: AIDS Education Policy and Young Women's Sexuality*. WRAP Paper 1. London, Tuffnell Press.

Holland, J., Ramazonoglu, C., Scott, S., Sharpe, S. and Thomson, R. (1990b) *Don't Die of Ignorance – I Nearly Died of Embarrassment: Condoms in Context*. WRAP Paper 2. London, Tuffnell Press.

Holland, J., Ramazonoglu, C. and Sharpe, S. (1993) *Wimp or Gladiator: Contradictions in Acquiring Masculine Sexuality*. WRAP/MRAP Paper 9. London, Tufnell Press.

Hollands, R.G. (1990) *The Long Transition*. London, Macmillan.

Huber, J. and Schneider, B.E. (eds) (1992) *The Social Context of AIDS*. London, Sage.

Hurrelman, K. (1990) 'Health promotion for adolescents: Preventive and corrective strategies against problem behaviour', *Journal of Adolescence*, 13, pp. 231–50.

Hurrelman, K. and Lösel, F. (1990) *Health Hazards in Adolescence*. Berlin and New York, de Gruyter.

Ingham, R. and Memon, A. (1990) *Methodological Issues in the Study of Sexual Behaviour in the Context of HIV Infection – an Overview*. Department of Psychology, The University, Southampton.

Ingham, R., Woodcock, A. and Stenner, K. (1992) 'Rational Decision Making Models and Sexual Behaviour', in Aggleton, P., Davies, P. and

Hart, G. (eds) *AIDS: Rights, Risk and Reason*, Lewes, Falmer.

Inhelder, B. and Piaget, J. (1958) *The Growth of Logical Thinking from Childhood to Adolescence*. London, Routledge and Kegan Paul.

Irwin, C.E. (1989) 'Risk-taking behaviour in the adolescent patient: are they impulsive?', *Paediatric Annals*, 18, pp.122–33.

Irwin, C.E. and Millstein, S.G. (1986) 'Biopsychosocial correlates of risk-taking behaviours during adolescence', *Journal of Adolescent Health Care*, 7, pp.825–965.

Ives, R. (1990a) 'Sniffing out the solvent users', in Ashton, N. (ed.) (1990) *Drug Misuse in Britain: National Audit of Drug Misuse Statistics, 1990*. London, ISDD.

Ives, R. (1990b) 'The fad refuses to fade', *Druglink*, 5, 5, pp.12–13.

Jack, M.S. (1989) 'Personal Fable: a potential explanation for risk-taking behaviour in adolescents,' *Journal of Paediatric Nursing*, 4, pp.334–38.

Jackson, A.E. (1987) *Perceptions of a New Acquaintance in Adolescence*. Groningen, Stichting Kinderstudies.

Jackson, A.E., Bosma, H.A. and Everts, P.A.A. (1990) 'Een ontwikkelingspsychologisch perspectiefop sociale vaardigheidstraining in de adolescentie' *Nederlands Tijdschrift voor de Psychologie*, 45, pp. 315–27.

Jeffs, T. and Smith, M. (eds) (1990) *Young People, Inequality and Youth Work*. London, Macmillan.

Jesson, J. (1993) 'Understanding adolescent female prostitution: A literature review', *British Journal of Social Work*, 23, pp.517–30.

Jessor, R. (1987) 'Problem behaviour theory, psychological development and adolescent problem drinking', *British Journal of Addiction*, 82, pp. 331–42.

Jessor, R. (1991) 'Risk behaviour in adolescence: A psychosocial framework for understanding and action', personal communication quoted in Plant, M. and Plant, M. (1992) *Risk-Takers, Alcohol, Drugs, Sex and Youth*. London, Routledge.

Jessor, R. and Jessor, S.L. (1977) *Problem Behaviour and Psychological Development*. New York, Academic Press.

Johnson, A.M., Wadsworth, J., Wellings, K. and Field, J. (1994) *Sexual Attitudes and Lifestyles*. London, Blackwell.

Jones, G. and Wallace, C. (1992) *Youth, Family and Citizenship*. Milton Keynes, Open University Press.

Jones, J. and Graham, H. (1992) 'Community development and research', *Community Development Journal*, 27, 3, pp.235–41.

Kar, S.B. Talbot, J. and Coan, C. (1986) 'Peers as health promoters among adolescents', *Education for Health*, 1, pp.37–44.

Kent-Baguley, P. (1990) 'Sexuality and youth work practice', in Jeffs, T. and Smith, M. (eds) *Young People, Inequality and Youth Work*. London, Macmillan.

207

Kirk, D. (1986) 'Health-related fitness as an innovation in the PE curriculum', in Evans, J. (ed.) *Physical Education, Sport and Schooling*. London, Falmer Press.

Kirk, D., Nelson, S., Sinfield, A. and Sinfield, D. (1991) *Excluding Youth: Poverty among Young People Living Away from Home*. Edinburgh Bridges Project and Department of Social Policy and Social Work, University of Edinburgh.

Kirkwood, G. and Kirkwood, C. (1989) *Living Adult Education: Freire in Scotland*. Milton Keynes, Open University Press.

Kitwood, T. (1980) *Disclosures to a Stranger*. London, Routledge and Kegan Paul.

Klee, H. (1991) 'Sexual risk among amphetamine misusers: Prospects for change'. Paper presented at the 5th Social Aspects of Aids Conference, London, March 1991.

Kleiber, D.A. and Rickards, W.H. (1985) 'Leisure and recreation in adolescence: Limitation and potential', in Wade, M. (ed.) *Constraints in Leisure*, Springfield, IL, C.C. Thomas.

Kohlberg, L. (1969) *Stages in the Development of Moral Thought and Action*. New York, Holt Rinehart & Winston.

Kroger, J. (1989) *Identity in Adolescence*. London, Routledge.

Kuhn, T. (1962) *The Structure of Scientific Revolutions*. Chicago, IL, University of Chicago Press.

Lerner, R.M. (1985) 'Adolescent maturational changes and psychosocial development: A dynamic interactional perspective', *Journal of Youth and Adolescence*, 14, pp.355–72.

Lerner, R.M. and Karabenick, S. (1974) 'Physical attractiveness, body attitudes and self-concept in late adolescents', *Journal of Youth and Adolescence*, 3, pp.7–16.

Levin, L.L. (1989) 'Health for today's youth: Hope for tomorrow's world', *World Health Forum*, 10, 2.

Lewin, C. and Williams, R.J.W. (1988) 'Fear of AIDS: the impact of public anxiety in young people', *British Journal of Psychiatry*, 153, pp.823–24.

Lewin, K. (1970) 'Field theory and experiment in social psychology', in Muss, R. (ed.) *Adolescent Behaviour and Society*. New York, Random House.

Lightfoot, J. and Marchant, J. (1990) *Involving Young People in their Communities*. Research and Policy Paper No 12. London, Community Development Foundation.

Lloyd, T. (1990) *Work With Boys*, Leicester, National Youth Bureau.

Long, S. (1991) 'Just as important as anybody else. An innovative health project aimed at and run by young women has opened in Manchester', *Health Matters*, 8.

Love, J.G. and Hendry, L.B. (1994) 'Youth workers and young participants: Two perspectives of youth work? *Youth and Policy*, (Special Issue, New Directions in Youth Work), **46**, pp.43–55.

Lye, E. (1988) 'No building, no power', *Youth in Society*, **142**, pp.17–18.

McDermott, D. and McBride, W. (1993) 'Crew 2000: Peer coalition in action', *Druglink*, **8**, 6, pp.13–15.

MacIntyre, S., West, D. and Ecob, R. (1989) 'West of Scotland Twenty-07 Study: Health in the community', in Martin, C. and McQueen D. (eds) *Readings for a New Public Health*. Edinburgh, Edinburgh University Press.

McKeganey, N.P. and Boddy, F.A. (1987) *Drug Abuse in Glasgow: An Interim Report of an Exploratory Study*. Report by Social Paediatric and Obstetric Research Unit, Glasgow, University of Glasgow.

McMullen, R. (1988) 'Boys Involved in Prostitution', *Youth and Policy*, **23**, pp.35–43.

McRobbie, A. and Nava, M. (1984) (eds) *Gender and Generation*. London, Macmillan.

McRobbie, A. (1991) *Feminism and Youth Culture*. London, Macmillan.

Magnusson, D. (1988) *Individual Development from an Interactional Perspective: A Longitudinal Study*. Hillsdale, NJ, Erlbaum.

Magnusson, D., Stattin, H. and Duner, A. (1983) 'Aggression and criminality in a longitudinal perspective', in van Dusen, K.T. and Mednick, S.A. (eds) *Prospective Studies in Crime and Delinquency*. Boston, Kluwer-Nijhoff.

Marcia, J.E. (1980) 'Identity in adolescence', in Adelson, J. (ed.) *Handbook of Adolescent Psychology*. New York, Wiley.

Marsh, A., Dobbs, J. and White, A. (1986) *Adolescent Drinking*. OPCS Social Survey Division, London, HMSO.

Marshall, S. and Borrill, C. (1984) 'Understanding the Invisibility of Young Women', *Youth and Policy*, **9**, Summer, pp.36–9.

Massey, D. (1990) 'School sex education: Knitting without a pattern?' *Health Educational Journal*, **49**, 3, pp.134–42.

Massimini, F. and Carli, J. (1988) 'The systematic assessment of flow in daily experience', in Csikszentmihalyi, M. and Csikszentmihalyi, I.S. (eds) *Optimal Experience*. Cambridge, Cambridge University Press.

Masterson, G. (1979) 'The management of solvent abuse', *British Journal of Adolescence*, **2**, pp.65–75.

Mayo, M. (1991) *Community Work into the Nineties*. Transcript of Speech at Concept Seminar, Moray House College.

Mays, V.M., Albee, G.N. and Schneider, S.F. (eds) (1989) *Primary Prevention of AIDS*. New York, Sage.

Meeus, W. (1989) 'Parental and peer support in adolescence', in Hurrelman, K. and Engel, U. (eds) *The Social World of Adolescents*. Berlin, de Gruyter.

Merchant, J. and Macdonald, R. (1994) 'Youth and the Rave Culture,

Ecstasy and Health, *Youth and Policy*, 45, pp.16–45.

Milburn, K. (1994) *Peer Education with Young People about Sexual Health: A Critical Review*. Working Paper. Edinburgh, Health Education Board for Scotland.

Moore, S. and Rosenthal, D. (1993) *Sexuality in Adolescence*. London, Cassell.

Morgan, M., Calnan, M. and Manning, N. (1985) *Sociological Approaches to Health and Medicine*. Beckenham, Kent, Croom-Helm (reprinted 1988 by Routledge).

MORI (1989) *Ten Years On*. London, MORI.

MORI (1990) *Young Adult's Health and Lifestyles*. Research conducted for Health Education Authority. London, MORI.

Morse, M. (1964) *The Unattached*. Harmondsworth, Penguin.

Mountain, A. (1990) *Lifting the Limits*. Leicester, National Youth Bureau.

Mountain, A. (1985) 'Making up for lost time'. *Youth in Society*. 101, pp.22–24.

National Curriculum Council (NCC) (1990) *Curriculum Guidance 5: Health Education*. York, National Curriculum Council.

Newcombe, R. (1991) *Raving and Dance Drugs: House Music Clubs and Parties in North-West England*. Liverpool, Rave Research Bureau.

Newcombe, R., Measham, F. and Parker, H. (1992) 'Drinking, drug taking and deviance among young people. Preliminary findings of the first stage of a longitudinal survey of 776 14–15 year olds in the North-West of England in 1991'. Paper presented at the *Health in Europe* Conference, University of Edinburgh. Alcohol and Offending Research Project, Department of Social Policy and Social Work, University of Manchester.

Nichols, A.K. and Mahoney, C.A. (1989) 'Fitness and activity evaluation in school children', in Health Promotion Research Trust, *Fit for Life: Proceedings of a Symposium on Fitness and Leisure*. Cambridge, Health Promotion Research Trust.

Nutbeam, D., Macaskill, P., Smith, C., Simpson, J. and Catford, J. (1993) 'Evaluation of two smoking education programmes under normal classroom conditions', *British Medical Journal*, 306, pp.102–06.

O'Bryan, L. (1989) 'Young people and drugs', in MacGregor, S. (ed.) *Drugs and British Society: Responses to a Social Problem in the Eighties*. London, Routledge.

O'Mahoney, J.F. (1986) 'Development of person description over adolescence', *Journal of Youth and Adolescence*, 15, pp.389–404.

Off the Record (1992) *Annual Report*. Stirling, Off the Record.

Oosterwegel, A. and Oppenheimer, L. (1990) 'Concepts within the self-concept: A developmental study on differentiation', in Oppenheimer, L. (ed.) *The Self-Concept: European Perspective on its Development,*

Aspects and Applications. Heidelberg, Springer-Verlag.

Orr, J. (ed.) (1987) *Women's Health in the Community.* Chichester, Wiley.

Ovenden, C. and Loxley, W. (1993) 'Getting teenagers to talk: methodological considerations in the planning and implementation of the Youth Aids and Drug Study, *Health Promotion Journal of Australia*, 3, 2, pp.26–30.

Palmonari, A., Pombeni, M.L. and Kirchler, E. (1989) 'Peer groups and the evolution of the self-esteem in adolescence', *European Journal of Psychology of Education*, 4, pp.3–15.

Paraskeva, J. (1991) 'The missing piece: the youth service should be a mandatory part of local authority provision', *Education*, 178, 12, p.231.

Pearson, G. (1987) *The New Heroin Users*, p.84. London, Blackwell.

Petersen, A.C., Ebatta, A.T. and Graber, J.A. (1987) 'Coping with adolescence: The functions and dysfunctions of poor achievement'. Paper presented at the Biennial Meeting of the Society of Research in Child Development, Baltimore, Maryland.

Peterson, C. and Stunkard, A. (1989) 'Personal control and health promotion', *Social Science and Medicine*, 28, 8., pp.819–28.

Pill, R, and Stott, N. (1985) 'Choice or change: Further evidence on ideas of illness and responsibility for health', *Social Science and Medicine*, 20, 10, pp.981–91.

Pintrich, P.R. Marx, R.W. and Boyle, R.A. (1993). 'Beyond cold conceptual change: The role of motivation beliefs and classroom contextual factors in the process of conceptual changes', *Review of Educational Research*, 63, pp.167–99.

Plant, M. and Plant, M. (1992) *Risk-Takers. Alcohol, Drugs, Sex and Youth.* London, Routledge.

Plant, M.A. and Stuart, R. (1984) 'The correlates of serious alcohol-related consequences and illicit drug use amongst a cohort of Scottish teenagers', *British Journal of Addiction*, 79, pp.197–200.

Prendergast, S. and Prout, A. (1987) *Knowing and Learning About Parenthood.* Cambridge Health Education Authority.

Ramsey, S. (1990) 'Dangerous games: UK solvent deaths 1983–1988', *Druglink*, 5, 5, pp.8–9.

Redhead, S. (1993) 'The end of the century party', in Redhead, S. (ed) *Rave off: Politics and deviance in Contemporary Youth Culture.* Aldershot, Avebury.

Redman, J. (1987) 'AIDS and peer teaching', *Health Education Journal*, 46, 4, pp.150–51.

Redman, J. (1988) 'Peer teaching in health education: Research into the potential of young people as educators in schools'. Unpublished MSc Thesis. Department of Health Education and Health Promotion, Leeds

Polytechnic.

Redman, J. (1992) *A Young Person's Health Project: What Do Young People in Dundee Want?* Dundee, Health Education Centre.

Redman, J. (1994) 'Bodymatters', *Xcellent: The Journal of Peer Education in Scotland*, 3. Edinburgh, Fast Forward Positive Lifestyles Ltd.

Redman, P. (1994a) 'Shifting Ground: Rethinking sexuality education', in Epstein, D. (ed.) *Challenging Lesbian and Gay Inequalities in Education*. Buckingham, Open University Press.

Redman, P. (1994b) 'Curtis Loves Ranjit: Coming to terms with pupils' sexual cultures'. Paper presented at British Sociological Association Annual Conference, University of Central Lancashire, 28–31 March.

Reid, D. (1981) 'Into the mainstream – a survey of progress and prospects', *Times Educational Supplement*, 17 April.

Rhodes, T. (1994) 'HIV outreach, peer education and community change: developments and dilemmas', *Health Education Journal*, 53, pp.92–9.

Rhodes, T., Holland, J. and Hartnoll, R. (1991) *Hard to Reach or Out of Reach: An Evaluation of an Innovative Model of HIV/Outreach Health Education*. London, Drug Indicators Project, Birkbeck College, University of London.

Rietveld, H. (1991) 'Living the dream: Analysis of the rave phenomenon in terms of ideology, consumerism and sub-culture'. Unpublished paper. Unit for Law and Popular Culture, Manchester Polytechnic.

Roberts, K. and Parsell, G. (1989) 'Recent changes in the pathways from school to work', in Hurrelman, K. and Engel, U. (eds) *The Social World of Adolescents*. Berlin, de Gruyter.

Roberts, K. and Parsell, G. (1990) 'Young people's routes into UK labour markets in the late 1980s'. ESRC 16–19 Initiative Occasional Paper No. 27. London, City University.

Rodriguez-Tomé, H. and Bariaud, F. (1984) 'Self-identity and self-knowledge in adolescence'. Paper presented at First European Conference on Developmental Psychology, Groningen.

Rodriguez-Tomé, H. and Bariaud, F. (1990) 'Anxiety in adolescence: Sources and reactions', in Bosma, H.A. and Jackson, A.E. (eds) *Coping and Self-concept in Adolescence*. Heidelberg, Springer-Verlag.

Rosen, G. and Ross, A. (1968) 'Relationship of body image to self concept', *Journal of Consulting and Clinical Psychology*, 32, p.100.

Rosenberg, M. (1979) *Conceiving the Self*. New York, Basic Books.

Rotherham-Borus, M.J., Becker, J.V., Koopman, C. and Kaplan, M. (1991) 'AIDS knowledge and beliefs, and sexual behaviour of sexually delinquent and non-deliquent (runaway) adolescents', *Journal of Adolescence*, 14, pp. 199–224.

Rutter, M. (1989) 'Pathways from childhood to adult life', *Journal of*

Child Psychology and Psychiatry, **30**, 1, pp.23–52.

Schofield, M. (1965) *The Sexual Behaviour of Young People*. London, Longman.

Schools Council (1977) *Schools Council Health Education Project 5–13*. London, Nelson.

Schools Council Health Education Project (1982) *Health Education 13–18 yrs: Co-ordinator's Handbook*. London, Forbes.

Scott, L. and Thompson, R. (1992) 'School sex education: More a patchwork than a pattern'. *Health Education Journal*, **51**, 3, pp.132–35.

Scottish Consultative Committee on the Curriculum (SCCC) (1990) *Promoting Good Health: Proposals for Action in Schools*. Edinburgh, HMSO.

Scottish Health Service Planning Council (1980) *Scottish Health Authorities Priorities for the Eighties*, (SHAPE). Edinburgh, HMSO.

Scottish Office Education Department (SOED) (1993) *Environmental Studies 5–14*. Edinburgh, HMSO.

Scraton, S.J. (1986) 'Images of femininity and the teaching of girls' physical education', in Evans, J. (ed.) *Physical Education, Sport and Schooling*, London, Falmer Press.

Sharp, D. and Lowe, G. (1989) 'Adolescents and alcohol – a review of the recent British research', *Journal of Adolescence*, **12**, pp.295–307.

Shaw, M. (1984) *Sport and Leisure Participation and Lifestyles in Different Residential Neighbourhoods. An Exploration of the ACORN Classification*. London, Sports Council.

Sheehy, G. (1976) *Passages: Predictable Crises of Adult Life*. New York, Bantam Books.

Shelter (1993) 'Trends in Youth Homelessness', *Scottish Housing Monitor*, **12**, pp.8–9.

Scottish Home and Health Department (SHHD) (1991) *Health Education in Scotland: A National Policy Statement*. Edinburgh, HMSO.

Shilts, R. (1988) *And the Band Played On*. London, Penguin.

Shucksmith, J., Philip, K., Francis, A. and Hendry, L.B. (1993) *Health Advice and Information Centres for Young People: An Investigation of Existing Alternatives*. Final report of a research project to Grampian Health Board. Aberdeen, Department of Education, University of Aberdeen.

Shucksmith, J., Philip, K. and Hendry, L.B. (1991) *Young People's Health: Lifestyles and Health Interventions in Community Settings*. Review of literature prepared for the Health Education Board for Scotland. Department of Education, University of Aberdeen.

Shucksmith, J., Philip, K. and Wood, S. (1995) *Peer Educators and Parent Collaborators, Report of an Action Research Study into Peer Education*. Aberdeen, Department of Education, University of

Aberdeen.

Sieniewicz, A. (1995) 'You have to give something of yourself: Two case studies of sex education programmes in Grampian schools'. Unpublished MEd thesis. Aberdeen, Department of Education, University of Aberdeen.

Silbereisen, R.K. and Noack, P. (1990) 'Adolescents' orientations for development', in Bosma, H.A. and Jackson, A.E. (eds) *Coping and Self-concept in Adolescence*. Heidelberg, Springer-Verlag.

Silbereison, R.K., Noack, P. and Eyferth, K. (1987) 'Place for development: adolescents, leisure – settings and developmental tasks', on Sillbererson, R.K., Eyferth, K. and Rudinger G. (eds) *Development as Action in Context: Problem Behaviour and Normal Youth Development*. New York, Springer-Verlag.

Simmons, R. and Rosenberg, S. (1975) 'Sex, sex roles and self image', *Journal of Youth and Adolescence*, 4, pp.229–56.

Smith, D.I. (1990) *The Numbers Game: Implications of the Changes in the Population of Young People for the Youth Service*. Leicester, National Youth Bureau.

Smith, M. (1988) *Developing Youth Work*. Milton Keynes, OUP.

Soper, D. (1993) 'The prophet in his own country', *Guardian*, 28 January, p.3.

Spence, J. (1990) 'Youth work and gender', in Jeffs. T. and Smith, M. *Young People, Inequality and Youth Work*. London, Macmillan.

Stacey, B. and Davies, J. (1970) 'Drinking behaviour in childhood and adolescence: an evaluative review,' *British Journal of Addiction*, 65, pp.203–12.

Stanworth, M. (1983) *Gender and Schooling*. London, Hutchinson.

Stattin, H. and Magnusson, D. (1990) *Pubertal Maturation in Female Development*. Hillsdale, NJ, Erlbaum.

Stears, D. and Clift, S. (1990) *A Survey of AIDS Education in Secondary Schools*. Horsham, Avert Trust.

Stegen, W. (1983) 'Sexual experience and contraceptive practice of young women attending a youth advisory clinic', *British Journal of Family Planning*, 8, pp.138–39.

Stein, M. and Frost, N. (1992) 'Empowerment and child welfare', in Coleman, J.C. and Warren-Adamson, C. (eds) *Youth Policy in the 1990s: The Way Forward*. London, Routledge.

Stewart, F. (1992) 'The adolescent as consumer', in Coleman, J.C. and Warren-Adamson, C. (eds) *Youth Policy in the 1990s: The Way Forward*. London, Routledge.

Streitmatter, J.L. (1985) 'Cross-sectional investigation of adolescent perceptions of gender roles', *Journal of Adolescence*, 8, pp.183–93.

Swadi, H. and Zeitlin, H. (1988) 'Peer influence and adolescent substance use: A promising side?' *British Journal of Addiction*, 83, pp.153–57.

Tajfel, H. (ed.) (1982) *Social Identity and Intergroup Relations.* Cambridge, Cambridge University Press.

Tanner, J.M. (1962) *Growth at Adolescence.* Oxford, Blackwell Scientific Publications.

Taylor, N. and Brierley, D. (1992) 'The impact of the law on the development of a sex education programme at a Leicestershire comprehensive school', *Pastoral Care*, 10, 1, pp.23–8.

Tayside Regional Council (1991) *Peer Education, a Briefing Paper*, 21st March.

Tayside Regional Council (1993) *Putting People First. A Policy Statement and Guidelines for Health Education and Health Promotion in the Context of Personal and Social Education.* Dundee, Tayside Regional Council Education Department.

Temple, S. and Robson, P. (1991) 'The effect of assertiveness training on self-esteem', *British Journal of Occupational Therapy*, 54, 9, pp. 329–32.

Thomas, D. (1983) *The Making of Community Work.* London, Allen and Unwin.

Tilford, S. (1991) 'Decision making skills and health education', *Journal of Health Education*, 29, 1, pp.10–16.

Tilford, S. (1992) 'Health matters', in Coleman, J.C. and Warren-Adamson, C. (eds) *Youth Policy in the 1990s.* London, Routledge.

Tobin, J.W. (1985) 'How promiscuous are our teenagers? A survey of teenage girls attending a family planning clinic', *British Journal of Family Planning*, 10, pp.107–12.

Tones, K., Tilford, S. and Robinson, Y. (1990) *Health Education: Effectiveness and Efficiency.* London, Chapman and Hall.

Travis, A. (1995) 'UK slated on children's rights failure', *Guardian*, 28 January, p.4.

Wadsworth, M. (1979) *Roots of Delinquency.* Oxford, Martin Robertson and Co. Ltd.

Wallace, C. (1989) 'Social reproduction and school leavers: A longitudinal perspective, in Hurrelman, K. and Engel, U. (eds) *The Social World of Adolescents.* Berlin, de Gruyter.

Wallerstein, N. (1993) 'Empowerment and health: The theory and practice of community change', *Community Development Journal*, 28, 3, pp.218–27.

Wallerstein, N. and Bernstein, E. (1988) 'Empowerment education: Freire's ideas adapted to health education', *Health Education Quarterly*, 15, 4, pp.379–94.

Wallerstein, N. and Sanchez-Merki, V. (1994) 'Freirian praxis in health education: Research results from an adolescent prevention program', *Health Education Research*, 9, 1, pp.105–18.

Walton, S. (1994) 'When children's rights are wrong', *Scottish Child*,

December.

Walton, S. (1995) 'When children's rights are wrong', *Scottish Child*, January.

Warren-Adamson, C. (1992) 'Dear Minister', in Coleman, J.C. and Warren-Adamson, C. *Youth Policy in the 1990s*. London, Routledge.

Watney, S. (1993) 'Emergent sexual identities and HIV/AIDS,' in Aggleton, P., Davies, P. and Hart, G. (Eds) *Social Aspects of AIDS: Facing the Second Decade*. London, Falmer.

Wellings, K. and Bradshaw, S. (1994) 'First heterosexual intercourse', in Johnson, A.M., Wadsworth, J., Wellings, K. and Field, J. (eds) *Sexual Attitudes and Lifestyles*, London, Blackwell, pp.68–109.

West, P. (1993) 'Do Scottish schoolchildren smoke more than their English and Welsh peers?' *Health Bulletin*, 51, 4, pp.230–39.

Whalen, A. (1994) 'Youth work and sexual abuse survivors', *Youth and Policy*, 46, Autumn, pp.56–60.

Whichelow, M.J. (1987) 'Dietary habits', in Cox, B.D. (ed) *The Health and Lifestyle Survey*. Cambridge, Health Promotion Research Trust.

White, P. (1991) 'Parents' rights, homosexuality and education', *British Journal of Educational Studies*, 39, 4, pp.398–408.

Whitehead, M. (1989) *Swimming Upstream: Trends and Prospects in Education for Health*. London, Kings Fund Institute.

Whyte, W.F. (1941) *Corner Boys: A Study of Clique Behaviour*. Indianapolis, Bobbs-Meriel.

Wight, D. (1990) *The Impact of HIV/AIDS on Young People's Sexual Behaviour in Britain: A Literature Review*. Working Paper No. 20. Glasgow, MRC, Medical Sociology Unit.

Wight, D. (1993) 'Constraints or cognition? Young men and safer heterosexual sex', in Aggleton, P., Davies, P. and Hart, G. (eds) *AIDS: The Second Decade*. Basingstoke, Falmer Press.

Williams, T., Wetton, N. and Moon, A. (1989a) *A Way In: Five Key Areas of Health Education*. London, Health Education Authority.

Williams, T., Wetton, N. and Moon, A. (1989b) *A Picture of Health. What do you Do that Makes You Healthy and Keeps You Healthy?* London, Health Education Authority.

Willis, P. (1977) *Learning to Labour: How Working Class Kids Get Working Class Jobs*. Farnborough, Saxon House.

Wodak, A., McArthur, T. and Carroll, T. (1990) 'Drugs and AIDS education for Australian youth: The get real project', *Hygie*, 10, pp.8–12.

Woodcock, A.J., Steaner, K. and Ingham, R. (1992) 'Young people talking about HIV and AIDS: Interpretations of personal risk of infection', *Health Education Research: Theory and Practice*, 7, 2, pp.229–47.

World Health Organization (WHO) (1977) *The Health Needs of Adolescents*. Geneva, WHO.

World Health Organization (WHO) (1982) *The Concepts and Principles of Health Promotion.* A summary report of the working group. WHO Regional Office for Europe, Copenhagen.

World Health Organization (WHO) (1986) *Young People's Health: A Challenge for Society. Report of a WHO Study Group on Young People and 'Health for All by the Year 2000'*, Technical Report Series 731, Geneva, WHO.

World Health Organization (WHO) (1986) *A Framework for Health Promotion Policy a Discussion Document, Health Promotion*, 1, pp.335–40.

World Health Organization (WHO) (1986) *Ottawa Charter for Health Promotion.* First International Health Promotion Conference.

World Health Organization (WHO) (1989) *The Health of Youth: Background Document Technical Discussion.* Geneva, WHO.

World Health Organization (WHO) (1989) *The Reproductive Health of Adolescence: A Joint WHO/UNFPA/UNICEF Statement*, Cited in Aggleton, P. and Kapila, M. (1992) 'Young People, HIV/AIDS and the Promotion of Sexual Health,' *Health Promotion International*, 7, 1, pp.45–51.

Wright, S.P. (1991) *Trends in Deaths Associated with Abuse of Volatile Substances 1971–1989.* London, St George's Hospital Medical School.

Wyness, M. (1992) 'Schooling and the normalisation of sex talk within the home', *British Journal of Sociology of Education*, 13, 1, pp.89–103.

Yates, K. (1994) 'Community development and community education'. Paper presented at the Scottish Community Development Conference, Falkirk, 11 May.

Young, I.M. (1991) 'Encouraging parental involvement in school,' in Nutbeam, D., Haglund, B., Farley, P. and Tillgren, P. (eds). *Youth Health Promotion: From Theory to Practice in School and Community.* London, Forbes Publications.

Young, S. (1994) 'Nine out of ten parents support sex lessons', *Times Educational Supplement*, 4 November.

Young Scot (1993) Issue No 17. Edinburgh, Scottish Community Education Council.

Youniss, H. and Smollar, J. (1990) 'Self through relationship development', in Bosma, H.A. and Jackson, A.E. (eds) *Coping and Self-Concept in Adolescence.* Heidelberg, Springer-Verlag.

Name Index

221

Subject Index